The *illustrated* lecture series

Nephrology, Electrolyte Pathophysiology and Poisoning

The *illustrated* lecture series

Neurology and Psychiatry	P. N. Plowman
Endocrinology and Metabolic Diseases	P. N. Plowman
Nephrology, Electrolyte Pathophysiology and Poisoning	P. N. Plowman
Haematology and Immunology	P. N. Plowman
Cardiology	T. J. Phillips, P. N. Plowman
Respiratory Medicine	P. N. Plowman
Alimentary Medicine and Tropical Diseases	P. N. Plowman, T. J. Phillips, S. J. Rose

In Preparation

Surgery

Anatomy

Obstetrics and Gynaecology

Pathology

Physiology

Ophthalmology

The *illustrated* lecture series

Nephrology, Electrolyte Pathophysiology and Poisoning

P. N. Plowman MA MD (Cantab) MRCP FRCR
Consultant Physician
St Bartholomew's Hospital and Medical College
London EC1 UK

MEDICAL EXAMINATION PUBLISHING COMPANY

Distributors in the United States & Canada:
Medical Examination Publishing Company
A Division of Elsevier Science Publishing Co., Inc.
52 Vanderbilt Avenue, New York, New York 10017

ISBN 0 444 01267 2

Printed in Great Britain

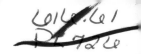

Contents

Preface

Renal diseases, the electrolyte and metabolic consequences of these disorders and their management have always proved a major stumbling block in the teaching curriculum of medical students and those paramedics involved with nephrology patients. However, given a simple explanation of nephron physiology and sites of damage, the consequences of disease may often be surmised from first principles or be easily understood and remembered.

The Illustrated Lecture Series has the major advantage in teaching this subject in that it provides a multitude of diagrams illustrating each key statement in the text. We believe that the many diagrams of the nephron demonstrating sites of damage and the sequelae in terms of poorly filtered, malabsorbed or inadequately secreted electrolytes, catabolites etc. will assist those in training to understand nephrology more simply.

It seemed logical to partner this subject with the primary abnormalities of fluid and electrolytes and also drug poisoning—a topic of contemporary importance and one relying on renal excretion and nephrological expertise. Lastly, the Chernobyl disaster has made us realise the importance of radiation poisoning, the fundamentals of which are discussed.

P. N. Plowman

Publisher's Note

Modern medicine is now more interesting and challenging than ever before. Unfortunately, the subject is now so large that it presents a formidable task for students to encompass and for the practising physician to maintain an up-to-date knowledge.

This series of illustrated books represents an entirely new concept which we believe will open up a new method of medical teaching, adding an extra dimension which will keep the reader's interest alive and active throughout the whole syllabus of general medicine.

The most important feature of the book is the linkage and locking of prose with figures in such a way that illustrations (with repeated key phrases) reinforce the comprehension of the text at all stages as one proceeds through the pages. The content of the series also differs from many standard works in that not only does it bring in new sections on subjects such as coma, brain death, blood transfusion reactions, etc. omitted in older texts, but it also recognises that certain diseases (e.g. tertiary syphilis) no longer merit extensive description whilst other subjects (e.g. current successes in oncology) merit a more generous coverage.

This series, when completed and collected together, should comprise a uniquely illustrated textbook for the entire medical curriculum. Although primarily intended for the undergraduate student, these books should also prove substantially helpful to nurses, paramedics and social workers who are academically inclined, and offer a refresher course to the busy practitioner.

We have tried to make academic life for the student easier. We shall welcome criticisms, comments and suggestions from academics, students and other readers since we feel sure that these will help us to improve future editions.

Nephrology

RENAL FUNCTION

The kidneys normally function to excrete waste products of metabolism (e.g. urea, creatinine, uric acid) and foreign chemicals (e.g. drugs) in the urine. The kidneys are the most important means by which the body maintains fluid and electeolyte homeostasis and this is achieved by varied volume and content of urine excreted. Lastly, the kidneys act as endocrine glands, secreting at least three important hormones: erythropoietin (a red cell, haemopoietic stimulant), 1,25–dihydroxycholecalciferol (the most potent vitamin D) and renin.

The functional renal unit is the "nephron" and there are approximately 1×10^6 nephrons per kidney. Each nephron is a thin tube $20 - 50\mu$ wide leading from the glomerulus in the renal cortex, eventually to end in the collecting duct in the

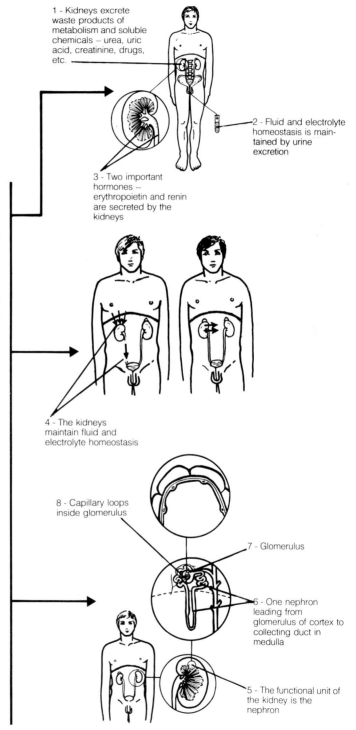

1 - Kidneys excrete waste products of metabolism and soluble chemicals – urea, uric acid, creatinine, drugs, etc.

2 - Fluid and electrolyte homeostasis is maintained by urine excretion

3 - Two important hormones – erythropoietin and renin are secreted by the kidneys

4 - The kidneys maintain fluid and electrolyte homeostasis

8 - Capillary loops inside glomerulus

7 - Glomerulus

6 - One nephron leading from glomerulus of cortex to collecting duct in medulla

5 - The functional unit of the kidney is the nephron

medulla. The **glomerular capsule** (Bowman's capsule) of each nephron envelops 4-6 capillary loops arising from an afferent renal arteriole. It is from these that the glomerular filtrate derives. Glomerular filtration is a passive process depending upon the hydrostatic pressure gradient between the blood and glomerular lumen; changes in blood pressure and flow changes in membrane permeability will affect the volume and content of the filtrate.

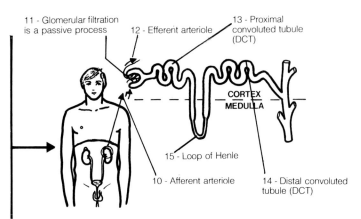

11 - Glomerular filtration is a passive process

12 - Efferent arteriole

13 - Proximal convoluted tubule (DCT)

CORTEX
MEDULLA

15 - Loop of Henle

10 - Afferent arteriole

14 - Distal convoluted tubule (DCT)

9 - The nephron comprises glomerulus, PCT, loop of Henle, DCT and collecting duct

The normal **glomerular filtrate** contains all plasma constituents at plasma concentrations (sodium, potassium, chloride, bicarbonate, urea, uric acid, creatinine etc) except plasma proteins and protein bound substances. In the **proximal convoluted tubule (PCT)**, glucose and amino acids are normally almost completely reabsorbed. Phosphate is actively reabsorbed from the PCT, (although under the inhibitory control of parathyroid hormone). Approximately 75 –80% of the sodium filtered by the glomerulus is reabsorbed from the PCT and chloride and water follow passively along the electrochemical gradient set up by sodium "pumping". Thus, approximately three quarters of the water and sodium filtered is reabsorbed in the PCT. Sodium reabsorption is linked to hydrogen ion excretion and bicarbonate reabsorption, (dependent on the renal tubular cell enzyme: carbonic anhydrase). The urine hydrogen ions are largely buffered by phosphates and ammonia but even so the urine pH may be as acid as 4.5. Potassium ions are almost completely reabsorbed by an active process in the **PCT**.

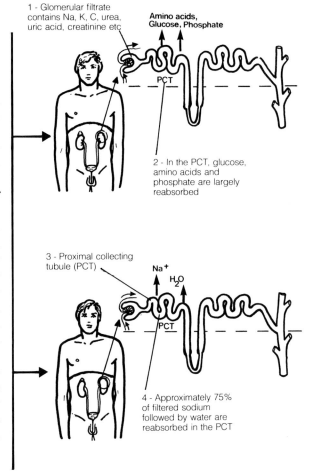

1 - Glomerular filtrate contains Na, K, C, urea, uric acid, creatinine etc

Amino acids, Glucose, Phosphate

PCT

2 - In the PCT, glucose, amino acids and phosphate are largely reabsorbed

3 - Proximal collecting tubule (PCT)

Na$^+$

H$_2$O

PCT

4 - Approximately 75% of filtered sodium followed by water are reabsorbed in the PCT

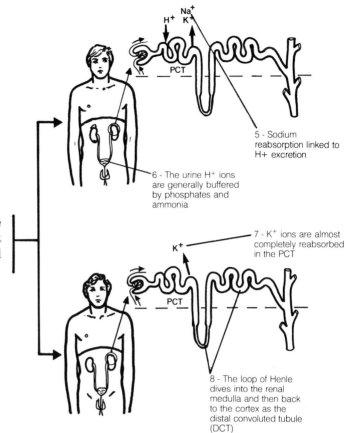

5 - Sodium reabsorption linked to H+ excretion

6 - The urine H+ ions are generally buffered by phosphates and ammonia

The **loop of Henle** dives down into the renal medulla and then comes back out again into the cortex to become the **Distal convoluted tubule (DCT)**.

7 - K+ ions are almost completely reabsorbed in the PCT

8 - The loop of Henle dives into the renal medulla and then back to the cortex as the distal convoluted tubule (DCT)

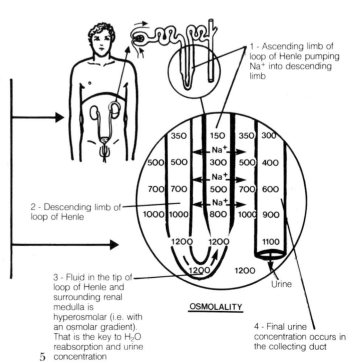

1 - Ascending limb of loop of Henle pumping Na+ into descending limb

In the loop of Henle, sodium is actively pumped from the ascending limb into the descending limb such that the fluid at the tip of the loop of Henle (and in the surrounding renal medulla) is hyperosmolar – an osmotic gradient is thus created in the renal medulla. It is this high osmolality deep down in the renal medulla that is the key to the final water reabsorption and urine concentration that occurs in the **collecting duct** as this too passes through the medulla.

2 - Descending limb of loop of Henle

3 - Fluid in the tip of loop of Henle and surrounding renal medulla is hyperosmolar (i.e. with an osmolar gradient). That is the key to H_2O reabsorption and urine concentration

OSMOLALITY

4 - Final urine concentration occurs in the collecting duct

Urine

5

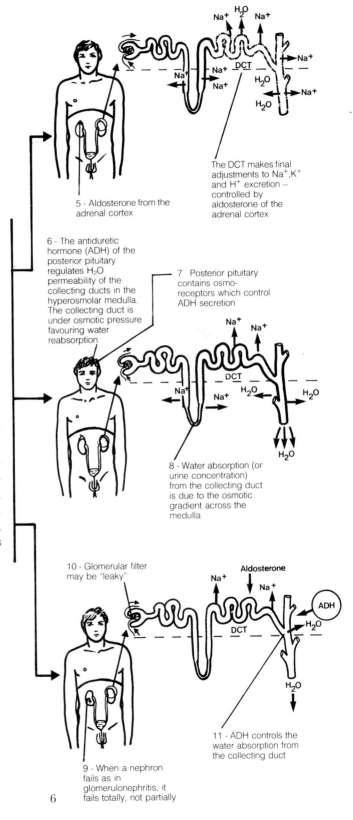

The DCT makes final
adjustments to Na^+,K^+
and H^+ excretion —
controlled by
aldosterone of the
adrenal cortex

5 - Aldosterone from the
adrenal cortex

6 - The antidiuretic
hormone (ADH) of the
posterior pituitary
regulates H_2O
permeability of the
collecting ducts in the
hyperosmolar medulla.
The collecting duct is
under osmotic pressure
favouring water
reabsorption

7 Posterior pituitary
contains osmo-
receptors which control
ADH secretion

8 - Water absorption (or
urine concentration)
from the collecting duct
is due to the osmotic
gradient across the
medulla

10 - Glomerular filter
may be "leaky"

11 - ADH controls the
water absorption from
the collecting duct

9 - When a nephron
fails as in
glomerulonephritis, it
fails totally, not partially

The **DCT** makes the final adjustments
to sodium, potassium and hydrogen ion
excretion, depending on the body's needs;
the hormone aldosterone stimulates
sodium reabsorption in exchange for
potassium at this site and carbonic
anhydrase is present in the **DCT** cells
also. The hormone: **Antidiuretic hormone** (ADH) regulates the water permeability of the collecting duct which, as
it passes through the hyperosmolar
medulla, is under osmotic pressure
favouring water reabsorption. The secretion of **ADH** from the posterior pituitary
is under the control of pituitary osmo-
receptors. Thus, the final urine composi-
tion is under fine control. In glomerulonephritis it is a feature that when a
nephron fails, it fails in toto and partial
nephron failure is not a feature; however,
tubular defects occur in other conditions
(see later).

TESTS OF RENAL FUNCTION

When considering defects in nephron function, the clinician needs to know if the glomerular filter is patent or deficient ("leaky") – and this is best screened for by the **colorimetric labstix** (urine analysis) for proteinuria; the normal urine protein excretion is less than 150 mg per day. The **glomerular filtration rate (GFR)** – giving a global view of overall nephron function – can be inferred to be low from the discovery of raised plasma urea and creatinine concentrations, but the GFR may have dropped somewhat before either of these values rise. A creatinine clearance, (derived from the 24 hour creatinine urinary excretion and the plasma concentration), gives a good working idea of **GFR**, if the urine collection is meticulously supervised. The direct measurement of **GFR** by the slope of plasma concentration decline after a single intravenous shot of chromium-51-labelled **EDTA** remains the most accurate assessment; (like inulin, this marker is freely filtered at the glomerulus but not reabsorbed by the tubules and thus excretion relates to filtration).

Urine Microscopy is a useful technique for quickly diagnosing urinary infection and detecting casts, red cells and crystals. It should be performed on unspun and centrifuged, fresh urinary specimens and viewed through a good binocular microscope. Casts imply renal pathology.

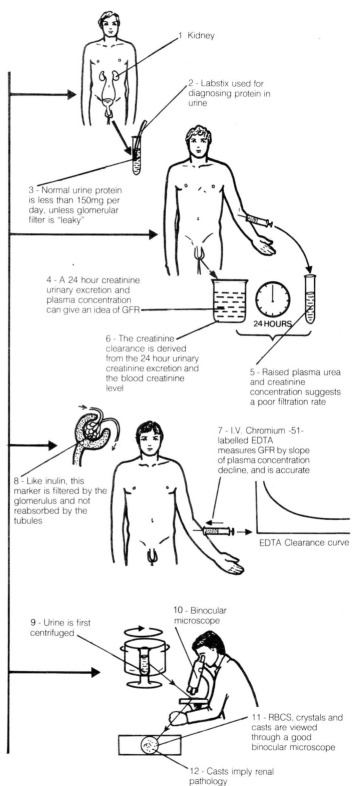

1 Kidney

2 - Labstix used for diagnosing protein in urine

3 - Normal urine protein is less than 150mg per day, unless glomerular filter is "leaky"

4 - A 24 hour creatinine urinary excretion and plasma concentration can give an idea of GFR

5 - Raised plasma urea and creatinine concentration suggests a poor filtration rate

6 - The creatinine clearance is derived from the 24 hour urinary creatinine excretion and the blood creatinine level

24 HOURS

7 - I.V. Chromium -51- labelled EDTA measures GFR by slope of plasma concentration decline, and is accurate

8 - Like inulin, this marker is filtered by the glomerulus and not reabsorbed by the tubules

EDTA Clearance curve

9 - Urine is first centrifuged

10 - Binocular microscope

11 - RBCS, crystals and casts are viewed through a good binocular microscope

12 - Casts imply renal pathology

The imaging of the urinary tract historically began with the **Intravenous urogram (IVU)**, the cystourethrogram and the retrograde pyelogram. **Nephrotomography**, **CT scanning** and **ultrasonography** have improved the imaging of the anatomical tract (and the last two techniques can be useful as they do not depend on function); **angiography** and radionuclide renograms have allowed us to determine blood flow and relative contributions to overall function by the two kidneys. However, the **IVU** remains the initial imaging technique in the assessment of urinary tract abnormalities. A routine IVU should be preceded by a series of plain abdominal films and the patient questioned concerning iodine hypersensitivity; an **anaphylaxis treatment kit** should always be available throughout the procedure. The **IVU** is usually performed with sodium salts of diatrizoate and following the bolus injection of 50 – 75 ml (15–20g iodine), the contrast is rapidly distributed throughout the extracellular space and promptly excreted by glomerular filtration – giving prompt **nephrogram** and slightly later pyelogram on X-ray.

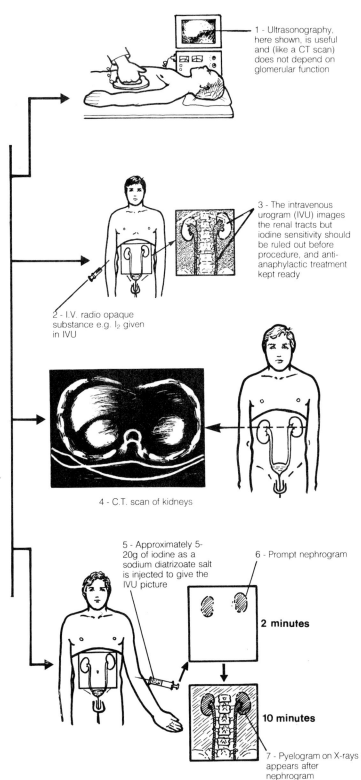

1 - Ultrasonography, here shown, is useful and (like a CT scan) does not depend on glomerular function

3 - The intravenous urogram (IVU) images the renal tracts but iodine sensitivity should be ruled out before procedure, and anti-anaphylactic treatment kept ready

2 - I.V. radio opaque substance e.g. I$_2$ given in IVU

4 - C.T. scan of kidneys

5 - Approximately 5-20g of iodine as a sodium diatrizoate salt is injected to give the IVU picture

6 - Prompt nephrogram

2 minutes

10 minutes

7 - Pyelogram on X-rays appears after nephrogram

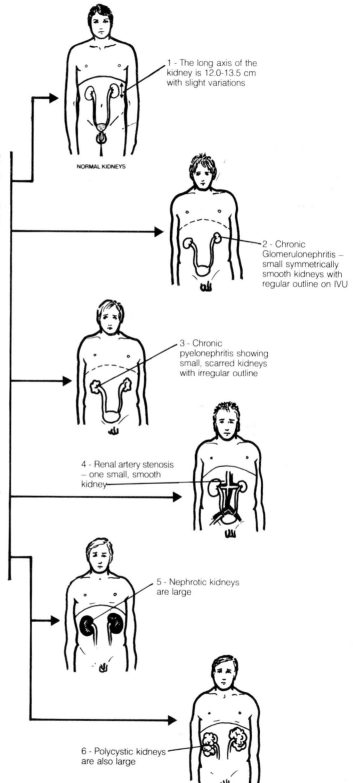

The normal adult kidney has a long axis of 12.0 – 13.5 cm, (approximately 3½ adjacent lumbar vertebrae), with a variation of not more than 1.5cm between the two kidneys. The common causes of **small kidneys** are:–

i) Chronic glomerulonephritis (small with regular outline on IVU; usually symmetrical). ii) Chronic pyelonephritis (small with irregular outline on **IVU**; often asymmetric). iii) Renal artery stenosis unilateral. The common causes of **large kidney(s)** on **IVU** are;– i) Nephrotic Syndrome. ii) Polycystic disease. iii) Hydronephrosis. iv) Unilateral hypertrophy following contralateral nephrectomy. v) Hypernephroma.

1 - The long axis of the kidney is 12.0-13.5 cm with slight variations

NORMAL KIDNEYS

2 - Chronic Glomerulonephritis – small symmetrically smooth kidneys with regular outline on IVU

3 - Chronic pyelonephritis showing small, scarred kidneys with irregular outline

4 - Renal artery stenosis – one small, smooth kidney

5 - Nephrotic kidneys are large

6 - Polycystic kidneys are also large

7 - Hydronephosis
increased size of
kidneys

In moderate renal failure, a higher dose of contrast injection can be used to obtain renal visualisation on IVU, but the contrast injection can precipitate acute-on-chronic renal failure when used in high dosage. Such patients should not receive more than 60g Iodine and should not be fluid restricted prior to **IVU**.

8 - Compensatory
hypertrophy following
surgery on fellow kidney

9 - Renal tumour e.g.
Hypernephroma
enlarges kidney

10 - Moderate renal
failure requires higher
dosage of contrast
injection for renal
visualisation on IVU but
this may further
damage kidneys

11 - More than 60g
Iodine should not be
given

The **radioactive renogram**, using **iodine–131**–Hippuran, gives a good overall measure of renal function with a comparison of the function of the two kidneys and gives an excellent demonstration of acute obstruction.

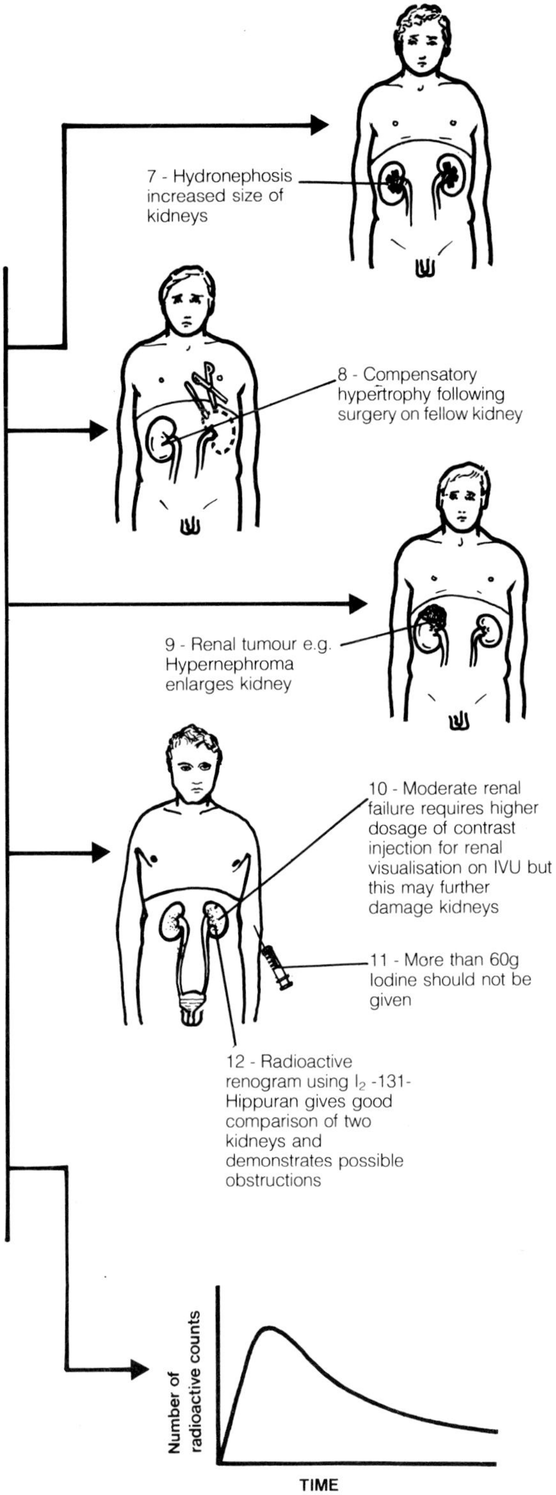

12 - Radioactive
renogram using I_2 -131-
Hippuran gives good
comparison of two
kidneys and
demonstrates possible
obstructions

Number of
radioactive counts

TIME
Normal Renogram Trace

Percutaneous renal biopsy is a most important means of obtaining a histological and immuno-histochemical diagnosis of renal parenchymal disease. However, it is not without hazard and there are specific indications: nephrotic syndrome, acute renal failure (not due to pre- or post- renal causes) and significant proteinuria (more than 1.5g per 24 hours). Prior to biopsy, the position of both kidneys should be known and both known to be functioning. Hypertension and uraemia should be under control and coagulation tests normal; blood should be ×-matched. The percutaneous biopsy is performed by a nephrologist and the patient rested in bed for 24 hours after the procedure, with frequent nursing observations.

ACUTE RENAL FAILURE

In **Acute renal failure (ARF)**, the kidneys' excretory and homeostatic functions become deficient and the urine output drops; (oliguria refers to a urine output of less than 400ml per 24hr. in an adult and anuria refers to absent urine flow). Urea creatinine and other waste products of protein metabolism accumulate in the blood and salt and water retention occurs; hydrogen ion excretion is deficient and hyperkalaemia often occurs. The situation may rapidly become life threatening.

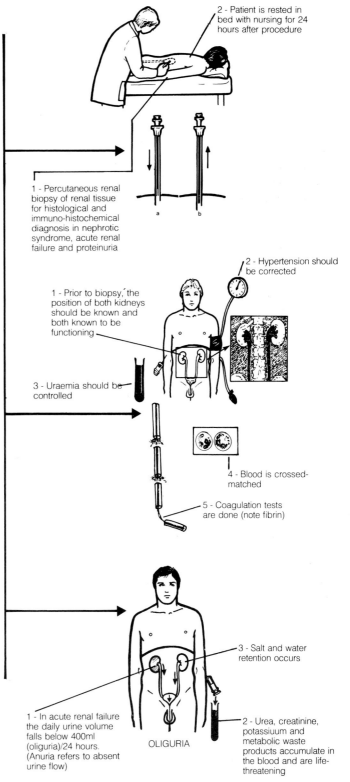

2 - Patient is rested in bed with nursing for 24 hours after procedure

1 - Percutaneous renal biopsy of renal tissue for histological and immuno-histochemical diagnosis in nephrotic syndrome, acute renal failure and proteinuria

a   b

2 - Hypertension should be corrected

1 - Prior to biopsy, the position of both kidneys should be known and both known to be functioning

3 - Uraemia should be controlled

4 - Blood is crossed-matched

5 - Coagulation tests are done (note fibrin)

3 - Salt and water retention occurs

1 - In acute renal failure the daily urine volume falls below 400ml (oliguria)/24 hours. (Anuria refers to absent urine flow)

OLIGURIA

2 - Urea, creatinine, potassiuum and metabolic waste products accumulate in the blood and are life-threatening

11

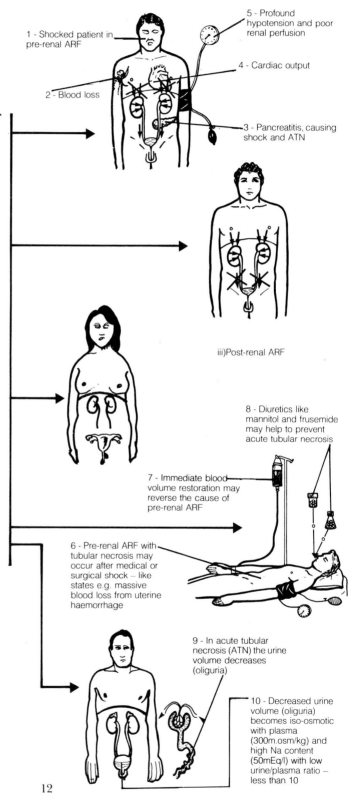

1 - Shocked patient in pre-renal ARF

2 - Blood loss

5 - Profound hypotension and poor renal perfusion

4 - Cardiac output

3 - Pancreatitis, causing shock and ATN

iii)Post-renal ARF

The now classic division of the causes of **ARF** into: Pre-renal, Renal and Post-renal **ARF**, still has many merits. **Pre-renal ARF** is the commonest form and is usually consequent upon blood loss, impaired cardiac output or septicaemic (or other e.g. pancreatitis) shock, all leading to profound hypotension and poor renal perfusion. Many medical, surgical and obstetric catastrophes may cause this prerenal shock and the renal ischaemia that follows leads to acute tubular necrosis (**ATN**) – the pathologic basis of pre-renal **ARF**. Rapid restoration of blood volume and reversal of shock may prevent **ATN** from occurring and the administration of diuretics - (e.g. mannitol, frusemide) early in the treatment of the shocked patient may also help to prevent **ATN**. Once **ATN** is established, the urine volume decreases (oliguria) and becomes isoosmotic with plasma (approx 300 m.OSM./Kg), containing an unusually high sodium concentration (more than 50mEq/l) and there is a low urine: plasma urea ratio, (less than 10). An **IVU** demonstrates dense nephrograms in **ATN** which persist for some hours; this demonstrates continued glomerular filtration.

8 - Diuretics like mannitol and frusemide may help to prevent acute tubular necrosis

7 - Immediate blood volume restoration may reverse the cause of pre-renal ARF

6 - Pre-renal ARF with tubular necrosis may occur after medical or surgical shock – like states e.g. massive blood loss from uterine haemorrhage

9 - In acute tubular necrosis (ATN) the urine volume decreases (oliguria)

10 - Decreased urine volume (oliguria) becomes iso-osmotic with plasma (300m.osm/kg) and high Na content (50mEq/l) with low urine/plasma ratio – less than 10

Hypercalcaemia and *hyperuricaemia* are two distinct pre-renal precipitants of ARF that should be screened for and quickly corrected. Hyperuricaemic ARF used to commonly follow treatment induction for acute leukaemia or lymphoma, but this is rare now due to prehydration and allopurinol adminstration.

11 - The IVU demonstrates dense nephrograms in Acute Tubular Necrosis (ATN) persisting for some hours indicating continued glomerular filtration

IVU

12 - Hypercalcaemia (left) and hyperuricaemia (right) are precipitants of ARF and should be quickly treated. Following treatment of leukaemia and lymphoma, hyperuricaemia develops unless this is prevented by prehydration and allopurinol

2 - In renal ARF there is no shock

1 - Renal ARF differs from pre-renal ARF. Indeed the patient may be hypertensive and this latter may accentuate renal ARF

4 - Drugs like Methicillin, aminoglycosides and Carbon Tetrachloride cause renal damage

5 - Acute glomerulonephitis and acute interstitial nephritis can be caused by drugs indicated above resulting in ARF

3 - Haemolytic uraemic syndrome is a rare cause of ARF

Renal ARF differs from prerenal **ARF** in that the patient does not present in hypotensive shock; indeed, the patients may be hypertensive and accelerated hypertension may predispose to renal **ARF**. Acute glomerulonephritis and acute interstitial nephritis (usually caused by drugs e.g. Methicillin) are the two commonest causes of renal ARF, but direct nephrotoxins (e.g aminoglycosides, carbon tetrachloride etc) form another group and the haemolytic uraemic syndrome is a further but unusual cause. An

6 - Early renal biopsy to diagnose acute glomerulonephritis and acute interstitial nephritis — common causes of ARF

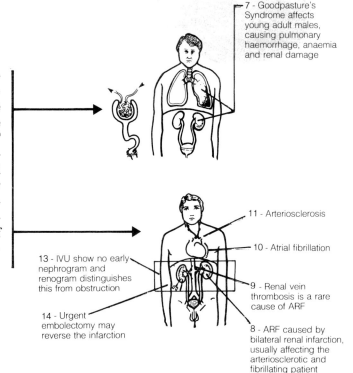

7 - Goodpasture's Syndrome affects young adult males, causing pulmonary haemorrhage, anaemia and renal damage

early renal biopsy is mandatory as thereby rapidly progressive (crescentic) glomerulonephritis, Goodpasture's syndrome and acute interstitial nephritis can be distinguished and treated. Renal **ARF** may be caused by bilateral renal infarction (usually in the arteriosclerotic and fibrillating); the **IVU** shows no early nephrogram and the renogram distinguishes this from obstruction – immediate embolectory gives the only chance of reversal. Renal vein thrombosis (bilateral) is a further rare cause.

11 - Arteriosclerosis

10 - Atrial fibrillation

13 - IVU show no early nephrogram and renogram distinguishes this from obstruction

9 - Renal vein thrombosis is a rare cause of ARF

14 - Urgent embolectomy may reverse the infarction

8 - ARF caused by bilateral renal infarction, usually affecting the arteriosclerotic and fibrillating patient

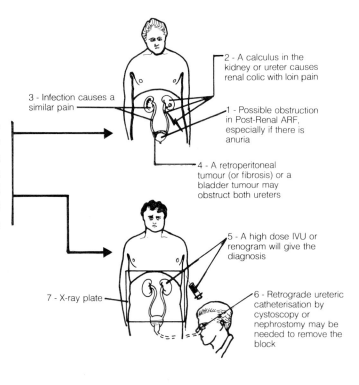

2 - A calculus in the kidney or ureter causes renal colic with loin pain

3 - Infection causes a similar pain

1 - Possible obstruction in Post-Renal ARF, especially if there is anuria

The possibility of obstruction (**post-renal ARF**) should be considered in every patient with **ARF** – particularly when there is anuria. When the cause is a calculus there is usually renal colic, and loin pains also feature when there are infected and obstructed kidneys; usually,

4 - A retroperitoneal tumour (or fibrosis) or a bladder tumour may obstruct both ureters

5 - A high dose IVU or renogram will give the diagnosis

7 - X-ray plate

6 - Retrograde ureteric catheterisation by cystoscopy or nephrostomy may be needed to remove the block

a retroperitoneal tumour (or fibrosis) or a pelvic (usually bladder) tumour may obstruct both ureters. A high dose **IVU** or renogram will give the diagnosis and cystoscopy with retrograde ureteric catheterisation or even nephrostomy may be needed to overcome the block.

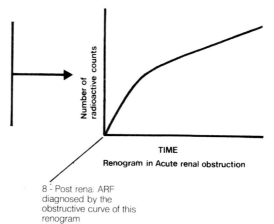

TIME

Renogram in Acute renal obstruction

8 - Post renal ARF diagnosed by the obstructive curve of this renogram

Management of ARF – Once ARF is established, the patient may be dehydrated or overhydrated and the simplest means of directly knowing the "day-to-day, state of play" is by the measurement of the central venous pressure (**CVP**) together with daily body weights. Accurate fluid balance is essential during ARF and the fluid intake requirement of an afebrile 70Kg adult is 500ml daily plus the daily volume of urine and other losses, (gut losses, burns area losses etc). In **ARF**, sodium depletion may occur out of proportion to dehydration and hypotension and reduced turgor together with a low plasma sodium suggest this. Hypernatraemia is uncommon without salt and water retention.

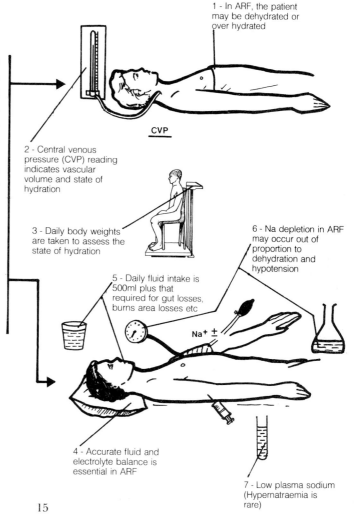

1 - In ARF, the patient may be dehydrated or over hydrated

CVP

2 - Central venous pressure (CVP) reading indicates vascular volume and state of hydration

3 - Daily body weights are taken to assess the state of hydration

6 - Na depletion in ARF may occur out of proportion to dehydration and hypotension

5 - Daily fluid intake is 500ml plus that required for gut losses, burns area losses etc

Na⁺ ±

4 - Accurate fluid and electrolyte balance is essential in ARF

7 - Low plasma sodium (Hypernatraemia is rare)

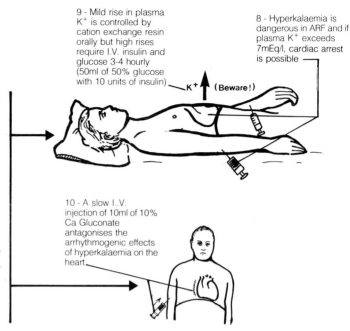

9 - Mild rise in plasma K$^+$ is controlled by cation exchange resin orally but high rises require I.V. insulin and glucose 3-4 hourly (50ml of 50% glucose with 10 units of insulin)

K$^+$ ↑ (Beware!)

8 - Hyperkalaemia is dangerous in ARF and if plasma K$^+$ exceeds 7mEq/l, cardiac arrest is possible

10 - A slow I..V. injection of 10ml of 10% Ca Gluconate antagonises the arrhythmogenic effects of hyperkalaemia on the heart.

Hyperkalaemia is a frequent and dangerous accompaniment of **ARF** – if the plasma potassium reaches or exceeds 7mEq/l, a cardiac arrest is possible. Lesser rises in plasma potassium are controllable by oral or rectal administration of a cation exchange resin but very high plasma potassium levels should be reduced by insulin and glucose intravenously, (50ml of 50% glucose with 10 units soluble insulin), repeated in 3 – 4 hours if necessary. A slow intravenous injection of 10ml of 10% calcium gluconate antagonises the arrhythmogenic effects of hyperkalaemia upon the heart.

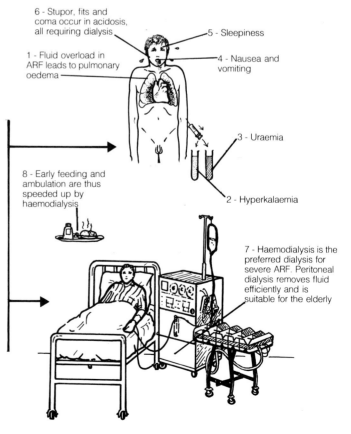

6 - Stupor, fits and coma occur in acidosis, all requiring dialysis

5 - Sleepiness

1 - Fluid overload in ARF leads to pulmonary oedema

4 - Nausea and vomiting

3 - Uraemia

2 - Hyperkalaemia

8 - Early feeding and ambulation are thus speeded up by haemodialysis

7 - Haemodialysis is the preferred dialysis for severe ARF. Peritoneal dialysis removes fluid efficiently and is suitable for the elderly

Patients with **ARF** and fluid overload, (usually presenting as pulmonary oedema), hyperkalaemia (plasma K+ 7.0mEq/l or more), uraemia (manifesting clinically with nausea vomiting, sleepiness, stupor, fits, coma) and acidosis – all require dialysis. Early and frequent **dialysis** maintains the patient in the best clinical condition. Although both peritoneal dialysis and haemodialysis are effective, haemodialysis is preferred in most centres as it allows early feeding and ambulation. Peritoneal dialysis remains a more efficient method of removing excess fluid and is better tolerated by the elderly.

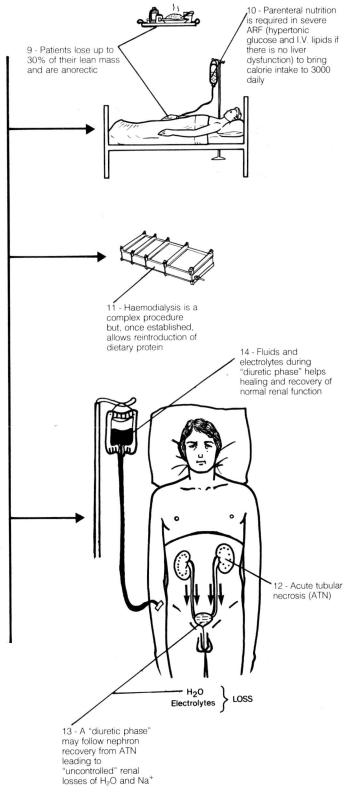

9 - Patients lose up to 30% of their lean mass and are anorectic

10 - Parenteral nutrition is required in severe ARF (hypertonic glucose and I.V. lipids if there is no liver dysfunction) to bring calorie intake to 3000 daily

11 - Haemodialysis is a complex procedure but, once established, allows reintroduction of dietary protein

14 - Fluids and electrolytes during "diuretic phase" helps healing and recovery of normal renal function

12 - Acute tubular necrosis (ATN)

H_2O
Electrolytes } LOSS

13 - A "diuretic phase" may follow nephron recovery from ATN leading to "uncontrolled" renal losses of H_2O and Na^+

Patients may lose up to 30% of their lean body mass during ARF and many patients are nauseated and unwilling to eat the low volume high calorie diet. Parenteral nutrition is required in most cases, concentrating on hypertonic glucose solutions and intravenous lipids, (unless there is hepatic dysfunction), to boost calorie intake to near 3000 calories daily. Once dialysis is established, protein may gradually be reintroduced along with some extra electrolytes.

The **outcome of ARF** is never certain and the overall death rate approaches 50% despite modern management methods. For patients with ATN who survive, then after one to three weeks of oliguria a "diuretic phase" occurs with uncontrolled renal loss of excessive amounts of water and electrolytes. It is very important to replace these losses during this "healing phase" and if fluid and electrolyte balance can be maintained, complete recovery of normal renal function will soon follow.

The **complications of ARF** are numerous but severe infections, (particularly Gram negative rod and staphylococcal septicaemias), and bleeding tendencies, (e.g. bleeding acute gastic ulcers), are the two commonest. The bleeding tendency is additional to the anaemia that is an inevitable accompaniment of renal failure.

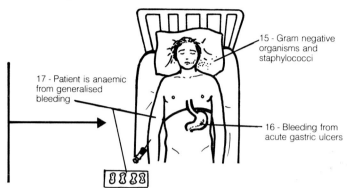

17 - Patient is anaemic from generalised bleeding

15 - Gram negative organisms and staphylococci

16 - Bleeding from acute gastric ulcers

GLOMERULONEPHRITIS

Glomerulonephritis refers to a spectrum of diseases, usually with an immunological basis, which cause damage to and dysfunction of the glomerular filtering membrane of all (or most) nephrons of both kidneys. This may lead to "acute glomerulonephritis", (with oliguria, haematuria, proteinuria, hypertension and perhaps severe ARF), or to "nephrotic syndrome", or over a period of time to chronic renal failure ("chronic glomerulonephritis"). Occasionally, recurrent symptomless haematuria occurs.

Acute Glomerulonephritis The syndrome of acute glomerulonephritis with the features just described may be caused by an acute streptococcal infection, (usually of throat or skin), or other infection, or as a complication of certain well-recognised systemic diseases viz: systemic lupus erythematosus (SLE), polyarteritis nodosa, **Henoch-Schoenlein purpura, Goodpasture's syndrome**. Occasionally, there is no identifiable predisposing medical condition.

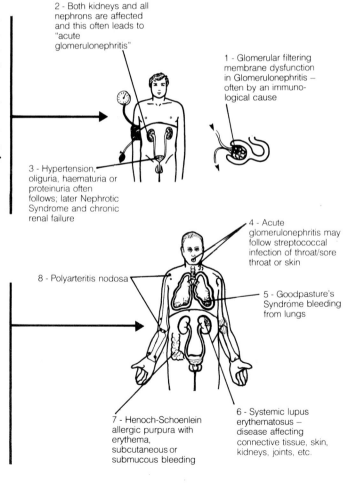

2 - Both kidneys and all nephrons are affected and this often leads to "acute glomerulonephritis"

1 - Glomerular filtering membrane dysfunction in Glomerulonephritis – often by an immunological cause

3 - Hypertension, oliguria, haematuria or proteinuria often follows; later Nephrotic Syndrome and chronic renal failure

4 - Acute glomerulonephritis may follow streptococcal infection of throat/sore throat or skin

8 - Polyarteritis nodosa

5 - Goodpasture's Syndrome bleeding from lungs

7 - Henoch-Schoenlein allergic purpura with erythema, subcutaneous or submucous bleeding

6 - Systemic lupus erythematosus – disease affecting connective tissue, skin, kidneys, joints, etc.

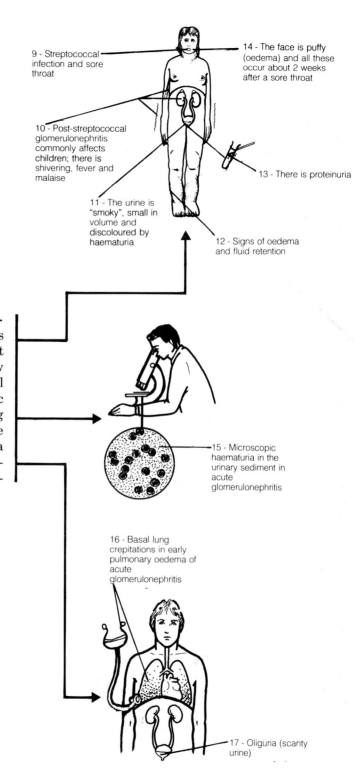

9 - Streptococcal infection and sore throat

14 - The face is puffy (oedema) and all these occur about 2 weeks after a sore throat

10 - Post-streptococcal glomerulonephritis commonly affects children; there is shivering, fever and malaise

13 - There is proteinuria

11 - The urine is "smoky", small in volume and discoloured by haematuria

12 - Signs of oedema and fluid retention

15 - Microscopic haematuria in the urinary sediment in acute glomerulonephritis

16 - Basal lung crepitations in early pulmonary oedema of acute glomerulonephritis

17 - Oliguria (scanty urine)

In **acute post-streptococcal glomerulonephritis**, which most commonly afflicts children, there is usually a fairly abrupt onset with malaise, shivering fever, puffy face (oedema), and "smoky" urine – (small volume, discoloured by microscopic haematuria and proteinuria), occurring approximately two weeks after a sore throat. On examination, there is oedema and occasionally other signs of fluid retention, (e.g. basal lung crepitations denoting pulmonary oedema), hypertension and oliguria. Urine microscopy demonstrates many granular and red cell casts.

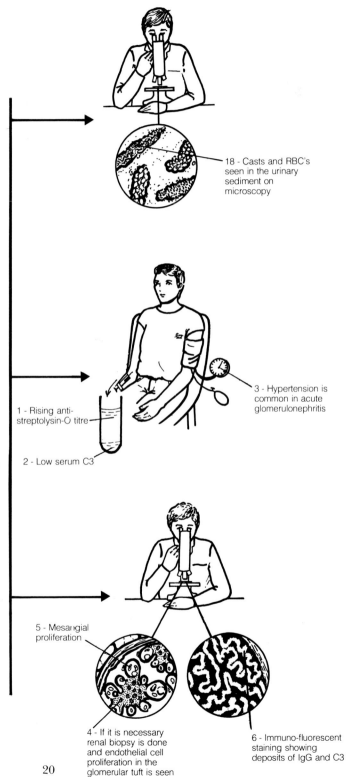

18 - Casts and RBC's seen in the urinary sediment on microscopy

Other **investigations** show a rising anti-streptolysin-O **(ASO)** titre and a low serum **C3,** (3rd component of complement). In such a case, it is rarely necessary to perform a renal biopsy. However, if biopsy were to be performed the uncomplicated case would show intense mesangial and endothelial cell proliferative glomerulonephritis, and immunofluorescent staining would show focal depositions of **IgG** and **C3.** The majority of children will recover spontaneously after a few days and conservative management, (i.e. quantified restriction) of fluid and electrolyte intake, together with a high calorie, low protein (20g protein daily) diet will usually obviate the need for dialysis. A diuresis usually occurs within a few days and heralds resolution. However, every case should be carefully monitored for the development of severe, anuric **ARF** requiring dialysis. It is wise to give penicillin to eradicate streptococci from the throat to all patients.

1 - Rising anti-streptolysin-O titre

3 - Hypertension is common in acute glomerulonephritis

2 - Low serum C3

5 - Mesangial proliferation

4 - If it is necessary renal biopsy is done and endothelial cell proliferation in the glomerular tuft is seen

6 - Immuno-fluorescent staining showing deposits of IgG and C3

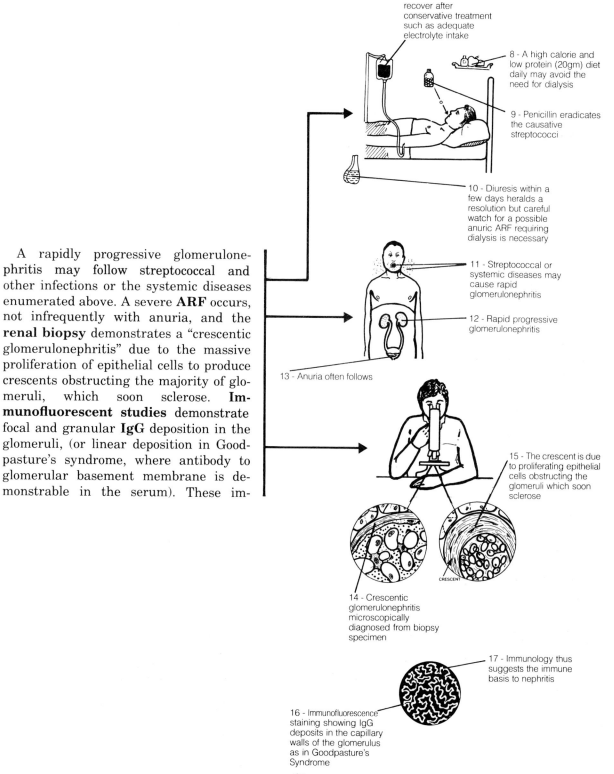

7 - Most children recover after conservative treatment such as adequate electrolyte intake

8 - A high calorie and low protein (20gm) diet daily may avoid the need for dialysis

9 - Penicillin eradicates the causative streptococci

10 - Diuresis within a few days heralds a resolution but careful watch for a possible anuric ARF requiring dialysis is necessary

A rapidly progressive glomerulone-phritis may follow streptococcal and other infections or the systemic diseases enumerated above. A severe **ARF** occurs, not infrequently with anuria, and the **renal biopsy** demonstrates a "crescentic glomerulonephritis" due to the massive proliferation of epithelial cells to produce crescents obstructing the majority of glo-meruli, which soon sclerose. **Im-munofluorescent studies** demonstrate focal and granular **IgG** deposition in the glomeruli, (or linear deposition in Good-pasture's syndrome, where antibody to glomerular basement membrane is de-monstrable in the serum). These im-

11 - Streptococcal or systemic diseases may cause rapid glomerulonephritis

12 - Rapid progressive glomerulonephritis

13 - Anuria often follows

15 - The crescent is due to proliferating epithelial cells obstructing the glomeruli which soon sclerose

CRESCENT

14 - Crescentic glomerulonephritis microscopically diagnosed from biopsy specimen

17 - Immunology thus suggests the immune basis to nephritis

16 - Immunofluorescence staining showing IgG deposits in the capillary walls of the glomerulus as in Goodpasture's Syndrome

munological data provide evidence for the immune basis to nephritis, (usually due to immune complex deposition in the glomeruli). Other histological "acute glomerulonephritic" appearances, both focal and diffuse, are recognised and, like crescentic/rapidly progressive glomerulonephritis, they are less likely to remit and have a more serious outlook than acute proliferative/poststreptococcal glomerulonephritis.

The **general management** of all acute nephritic cases comprises adequate nutrition (but low in protein) and obsessional control over fluid and electrolyte intake. Diuretics (usually Frusemide) and antihypertensives (Propranolol and, if necessary Hydralazine) may be required. The indications for dialysis are: i) Volume overload. ii) Hyperkalaemia. iii) Blood urea 60 mmol/l and creatinine 800 μmol/l.

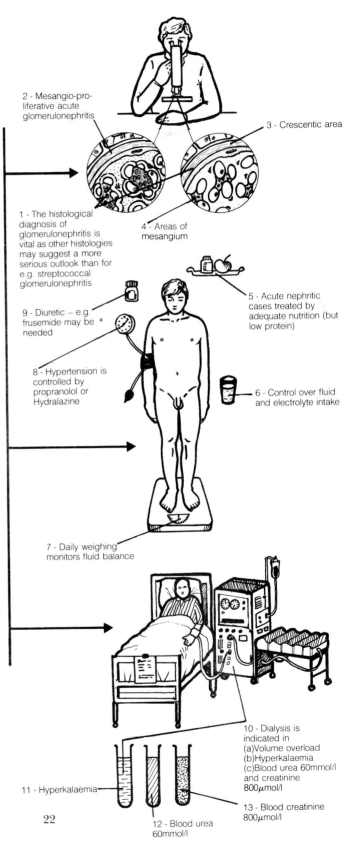

2 - Mesangio-proliferative acute glomerulonephritis

3 - Crescentic area

1 - The histological diagnosis of glomerulonephritis is vital as other histologies may suggest a more serious outlook than for e.g. streptococcal glomerulonephritis

4 - Areas of mesangium

5 - Acute nephritic cases treated by adequate nutrition (but low protein)

9 - Diuretic – e.g. frusemide may be needed

8 - Hypertension is controlled by propranolol or Hydralazine

6 - Control over fluid and electrolyte intake

7 - Daily weighing monitors fluid balance

10 - Dialysis is indicated in (a)Volume overload (b)Hyperkalaemia (c)Blood urea 60mmol/l and creatinine 800μmol/l

11 - Hyperkalaemia

13 - Blood creatinine 800μmol/l

12 - Blood urea 60mmol/l

Specific therapy for acute glomerulonephritis remains controversial. High dose steroids sometimes supplemented with cyclophosphamide (as an immunosuppressant) and heparin plus dipyridamole have been demonstrated to be useful in lupus nephritis and some other rapidly progressive glomerulonephritides. Plasma exchange (plasmapheresis) has proved useful in Goodpasture's syndrome (where it removes the antibody) and some crescentic/rapidly progressive cases, (probably due to removal of immune complexes). In general, if the glomerulonephritis does not rapidly come under control, it may be best to accept the irreversibility of the condition and plan a dialysis programme.

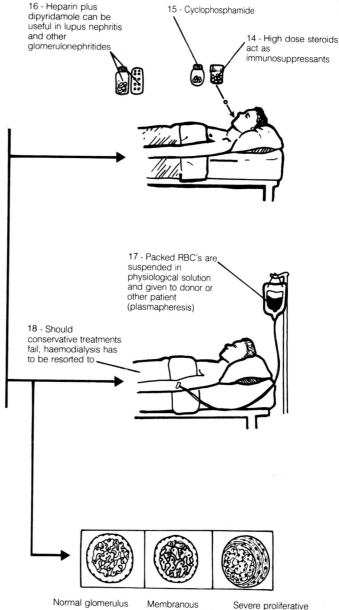

16 - Heparin plus dipyridamole can be useful in lupus nephritis and other glomerulonephritides

15 - Cyclophosphamide

14 - High dose steroids act as immunosuppressants

17 - Packed RBC's are suspended in physiological solution and given to donor or other patient (plasmapheresis)

18 - Should conservative treatments fail, haemodialysis has to be resorted to

Normal glomerulus

Membranous glomerulonephritis

Severe proliferative glomerulonephritis with crescent

THE NEPHROTIC SYNDROME

The normal person does not excrete more than 150mg protein in the urine per day and the colorimetic urine testing sticks (e.g Albustix) which reads "trace positive" at 4mg albumin per 100ml urine, usually records a negative. Some individuals may demonstrate transient, light proteinuria – for example during a fever. Patients with hypertension or cardiovascular disease may have proteinuria

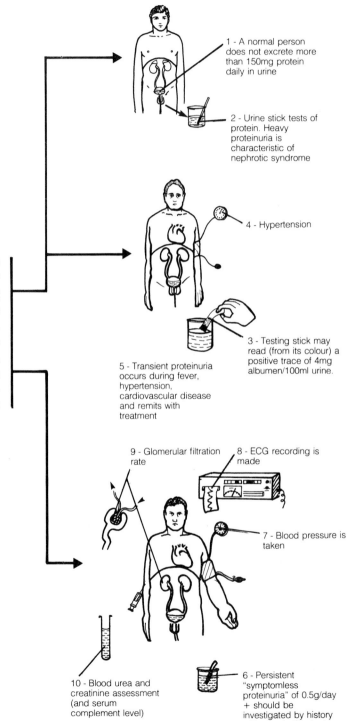

1 - A normal person does not excrete more than 150mg protein daily in urine

2 - Urine stick tests of protein. Heavy proteinuria is characteristic of nephrotic syndrome

4 - Hypertension

3 - Testing stick may read (from its colour) a positive trace of 4mg albumen/100ml urine.

5 - Transient proteinuria occurs during fever, hypertension, cardiovascular disease and remits with treatment

9 - Glomerular filtration rate

8 - ECG recording is made

7 - Blood pressure is taken

10 - Blood urea and creatinine assessment (and serum complement level)

6 - Persistent "symptomless proteinuria" of 0.5g/day + should be investigated by history taking and other tests

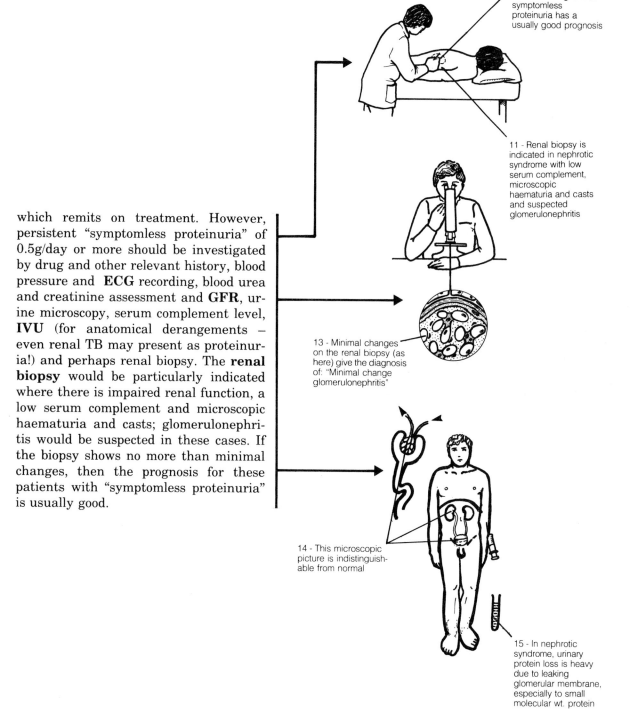

12 - Biopsy showing minimal changes with symptomless proteinuria has a usually good prognosis

11 - Renal biopsy is indicated in nephrotic syndrome with low serum complement, microscopic haematuria and casts and suspected glomerulonephritis

13 - Minimal changes on the renal biopsy (as here) give the diagnosis of: "Minimal change glomerulonephritis"

14 - This microscopic picture is indistinguishable from normal

15 - In nephrotic syndrome, urinary protein loss is heavy due to leaking glomerular membrane, especially to small molecular wt. protein

which remits on treatment. However, persistent "symptomless proteinuria" of 0.5g/day or more should be investigated by drug and other relevant history, blood pressure and **ECG** recording, blood urea and creatinine assessment and **GFR**, urine microscopy, serum complement level, **IVU** (for anatomical derangements — even renal TB may present as proteinuria!) and perhaps renal biopsy. The **renal biopsy** would be particularly indicated where there is impaired renal function, a low serum complement and microscopic haematuria and casts; glomerulonephritis would be suspected in these cases. If the biopsy shows no more than minimal changes, then the prognosis for these patients with "symptomless proteinuria" is usually good.

In the nephrotic syndrome, the urinary protein loss is heavy and this leads secondarily to hypoalbuminaemia and oedema. The pathological basis to the nephrotic syndrome is a damaged and leaking glomerular membrane – more "leaky" to small molecular weight protein (e.g albumen) than large molecular weight protein (e.g. globulin). Indeed, measurement of the protein leak profile (differential protein clearance) to some extent characterises the glomerular damage. Hypoalbuminaemia usually occurs when the urinary protein loss is greater than 3g/day, (and in severe cases of nephrosis may be up to 20g/day). The hypoalbuminaemia leads to a fall in the colloid osmotic pressure in the blood and this allows accumulation of fluid in tissue spaces. The fall in blood volume causes secondary hyperaldosteronism and the aldosterone secreted causes more salt (and water) retention, exacerbating the oedema. Another parallel change in the blood is a rise in plasma cholesterol and triglycerides.

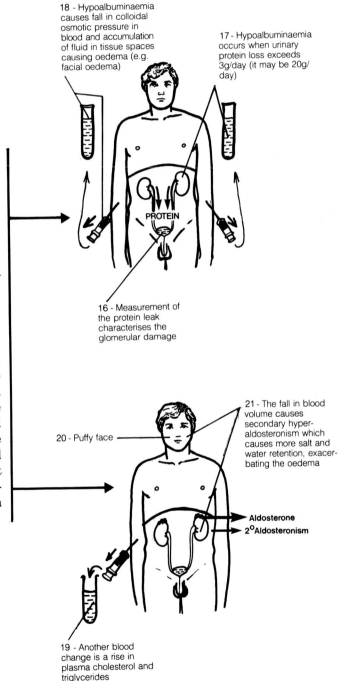

18 - Hypoalbuminaemia causes fall in colloidal osmotic pressure in blood and accumulation of fluid in tissue spaces causing oedema (e.g. facial oedema)

17 - Hypoalbuminaemia occurs when urinary protein loss exceeds 3g/day (it may be 20g/day)

PROTEIN

16 - Measurement of the protein leak characterises the glomerular damage

20 - Puffy face

21 - The fall in blood volume causes secondary hyperaldosteronism which causes more salt and water retention, exacerbating the oedema

Aldosterone
2°Aldosteronism

19 - Another blood change is a rise in plasma cholesterol and triglycerides

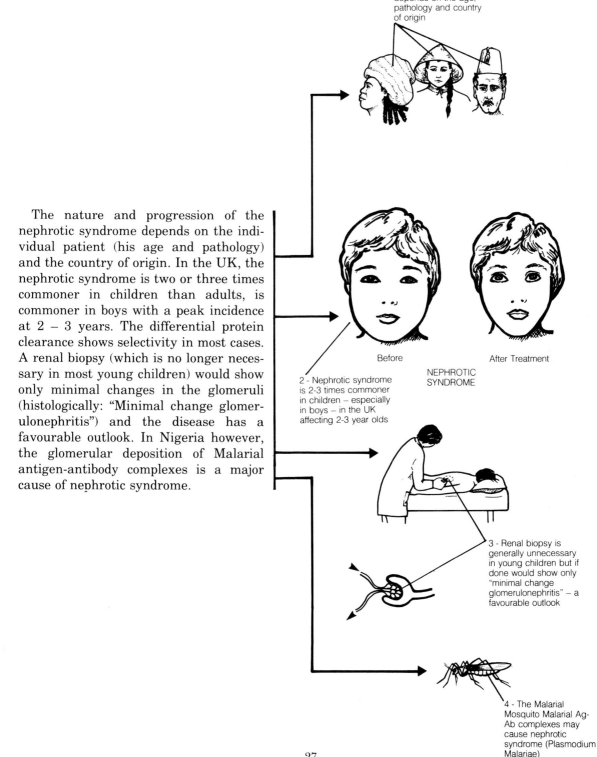

1 - The nature and progression of nephrotic syndrome depends on the age, pathology and country of origin

The nature and progression of the nephrotic syndrome depends on the individual patient (his age and pathology) and the country of origin. In the UK, the nephrotic syndrome is two or three times commoner in children than adults, is commoner in boys with a peak incidence at 2 – 3 years. The differential protein clearance shows selectivity in most cases. A renal biopsy (which is no longer necessary in most young children) would show only minimal changes in the glomeruli (histologically: "Minimal change glomerulonephritis") and the disease has a favourable outlook. In Nigeria however, the glomerular deposition of Malarial antigen-antibody complexes is a major cause of nephrotic syndrome.

Before   After Treatment

NEPHROTIC SYNDROME

2 - Nephrotic syndrome is 2-3 times commoner in children – especially in boys – in the UK affecting 2-3 year olds

3 - Renal biopsy is generally unnecessary in young children but if done would show only "minimal change glomerulonephritis" – a favourable outlook

4 - The Malarial Mosquito Malarial Ag-Ab complexes may cause nephrotic syndrome (Plasmodium Malariae)

In older children and adults nephrotic syndrome is usually more serious, (although minimal change histology is still the cause in 20%), and renal biopsy is usually an essential investigation. Proliferative glomerulonephritis is a common histological description in these cases; in the good prognosis post-streptococcal cases described above, the proteinuria usually subsides with time and it is the nephritic picture which presents. It is also the nephritic picture which tends to present in the rapidly progressive, crescentic glomerulonephritis, e.g. accompanying systemic lupus erythematosus **(SLE),** although the protein leak may be substantial and the nephrotic picture may sometimes dominate the presentation.

A common **histological picture** amongst patients with idiopathic nephrotic syndrome is: diffuse mesangial proliferative glomerulonephritis – where IgA deposits are commonly demonstrable; the progression is capricious.

5 - *In older children and adults, nephrotic syndrome is more serious (even with minimal change in biopsy) and biopsy is essential

6 - In post-streptococcal cases, however, the proteinuria subsides, the nephritic picture presents and the prognosis is good

7 - Thrombosis often develops in capillaries

8 - Capillaries in the glomerular tuft

9 - Fibrous crescents form squeezing the capillaries until the whole tuft is fibrosed

10 - Increase in mesangial cells where IgA deposits are demonstrable

11 - Capillaries are progressively narrrowed

12 - Proliferative glomerulonephritis may cause nephrotic syndrome. If this progresses to crescentic nephritis, the prognosis is worse

Membranous glomerulonephritis is another and interesting cause of nephrotic syndrome in which subendothelial deposits of immune complexes are demonstrable. The complexes appear enveloped by thickened basement membrane which, under the

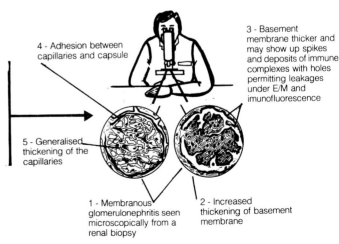

4 - Adhesion between capillaries and capsule

3 - Basement membrane thicker and may show up spikes and deposits of immune complexes with holes permitting leakages under E/M and imunofluorescence

5 - Generalised thickening of the capillaries

1 - Membranous glomerulonephritis seen microscopically from a renal biopsy

2 - Increased thickening of basement membrane

electron microscope appears to have ragged holes – accounting for the leak. This condition may be idiopathic or accompany connective tissue disorders, (e.g. SLE, rheumatoid disease) or some malignancies (e.g. carcinoma of bronchus, Hodgkin's disease). Certain infections (e.g. malaria, syphilis, hepatitis B, filariasis, leprosy) may cause membranous nephropathy and also certain drugs (e.g. gold, penicillamine, tolbutamide). These patients present with nephrotic syndrome and only a minority have macroscopic haematuria, hypertension or impaired renal function; hypocomplementaemia is not a feature.

Other histological patterns are well-recognised in association with the nephrotic syndrome (e.g. focal glomerulosclerosis) and when the nephrotic syndrome occurs during the course of some systemic diseases (e.g. amyloidosis, diabetics mellitus), the glomerular histology may be highly typical for that disease.

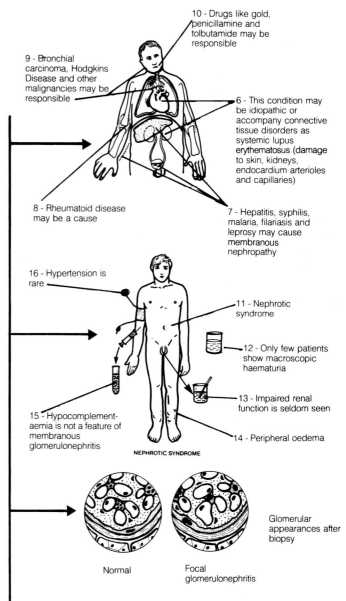

10 - Drugs like gold, penicillamine and tolbutamide may be responsible

9 - Bronchial carcinoma, Hodgkins Disease and other malignancies may be responsible

6 - This condition may be idiopathic or accompany connective tissue disorders as systemic lupus erythematosus (damage to skin, kidneys, endocardium arterioles and capillaries)

8 - Rheumatoid disease may be a cause

7 - Hepatitis, syphilis, malaria, filariasis and leprosy may cause membranous nephropathy

16 - Hypertension is rare

11 - Nephrotic syndrome

12 - Only few patients show macroscopic haematuria

13 - Impaired renal function is seldom seen

15 - Hypocomplementaemia is not a feature of membranous glomerulonephritis

14 - Peripheral oedema

NEPHROTIC SYNDROME

Glomerular appearances after biopsy

Normal

Focal glomerulonephritis

29

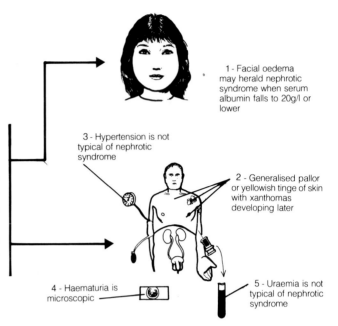

The **clinical onset** of nephrotic synrome is usually insidious with the gradual onset of dependent and facial oedema (which occur once the serum albumin has fallen to 20g/l or lower) and generalised pallor, (with perhaps a yellowish tinge to the skin and later xanthomas developing). Hypertension and uraemia are not features of the nephrotic syndrome per se and any haematuria is frequently microscopic.

1 - Facial oedema may herald nephrotic syndrome when serum albumin falls to 20g/l or lower

3 - Hypertension is not typical of nephrotic syndrome

2 - Generalised pallor or yellowish tinge of skin with xanthomas developing later

4 - Haematuria is microscopic

5 - Uraemia is not typical of nephrotic syndrome

The most important clinical distinction to be made is to detect those patients with "minimal change nephritis" from the other groups. Young children are very likely to have minimal change disease unless they have one or more of the following:– i) Haematuria. ii) Hypertension. iii) Hypocomplementaemia. iv) Reduced GFR v) Non-selective differential protein clearances. These features should be regarded as indications for a renal biopsy. The histological features seen on the renal biopsy specimen will usually allow the nephrologist to give a prognosis and sometimes assist in the specific treatment.

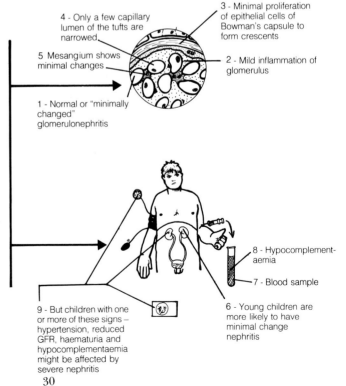

4 - Only a few capillary lumen of the tufts are narrowed

3 - Minimal proliferation of epithelial cells of Bowman's capsule to form crescents

5 Mesangium shows minimal changes

2 - Mild inflammation of glomerulus

1 - Normal or "minimally changed" glomerulonephritis

8 - Hypocomplementaemia

7 - Blood sample

6 - Young children are more likely to have minimal change nephritis

9 - But children with one or more of these signs – hypertension, reduced GFR, haematuria and hypocomplementaemia might be affected by severe nephritis

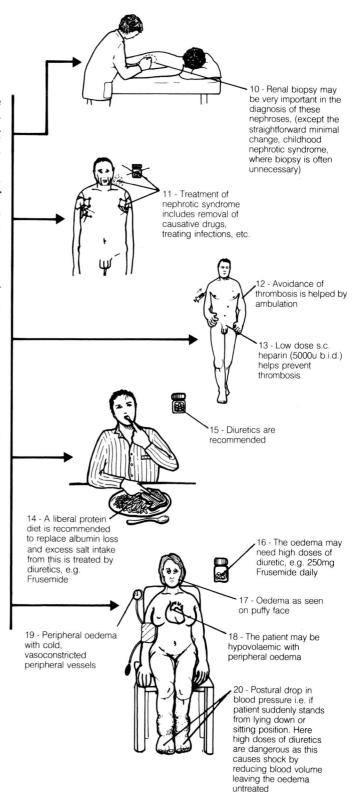

The treatment of nephrotic syndrome comprises firstly the removal or treatment of any underlying and precipitating condition (e.g drug causes, infections, Hodgkin's disease etc). Secondly comes the symptomatic treatment. Here it is important to keep the patient ambulant if possible, to avoid thrombosis, and as there is a coagulation tendency in nephrotic syndrome, many physicians recommend low dose subcutaneous heparin (5000u b.d.) as a matter of routine. Protein malnutrition is another concomitant of nephrotic syndrome and a liberal dietary intake of animal protein is recommended; this only partially ameliorates the problem of albumin loss, hepatic production being finite. The protein intake will be accompanied by extra salt intake, but this is usually not a problem as salt balance can usually be controlled by diuretics (e.g. Frusemide). Sometimes the oedema requires high doses of diuretic, (e.g. Frusemide 250mg daily) for a response. On other occasions, the patient may be **hypovolaemic** with peripheral oedema – the key physical signs of hypovolaemia being a cold, vasoconstricted periphery and a postural drop in the blood pressure. In this last circumstance, it would be dangerous to give large doses of diuretic as this would reduce the blood volume further, (creating a shocked patient), without reducing the oedema. The **manage-**

10 - Renal biopsy may be very important in the diagnosis of these nephroses, (except the straightforward minimal change, childhood nephrotic syndrome, where biopsy is often unnecessary)

11 - Treatment of nephrotic syndrome includes removal of causative drugs, treating infections, etc.

12 - Avoidance of thrombosis is helped by ambulation

13 - Low dose s.c. heparin (5000u b.i.d.) helps prevent thrombosis

15 - Diuretics are recommended

14 - A liberal protein diet is recommended to replace albumin loss and excess salt intake from this is treated by diuretics, e.g. Frusemide

16 - The oedema may need high doses of diuretic, e.g. 250mg Frusemide daily

17 - Oedema as seen on puffy face

19 - Peripheral oedema with cold, vasoconstricted peripheral vessels

18 - The patient may be hypovolaemic with peripheral oedema

20 - Postural drop in blood pressure i.e. if patient suddenly stands from lying down or sitting position. Here high doses of diuretics are dangerous as this causes shock by reducing blood volume leaving the oedema untreated

1 - I.V. Infusion of plasma of salt-free albumin and diuretic is the management of oedema and hypovolaemia

2 - Prophylactic penicillin reduces the risk of sepsis

ment of such patients is by the combined intravenous infusion of plasma or salt-free albumin and diuretic. Very oedematous patients are placed on prophylactic penicillin as they are at risk of sepsis.

With regard to **specific treatment**, it is quite clear that corticosteroids should be used to treat minimal change "glomerulonephritis" causing nephrotic syndrome. **Treatment** is commenced with 60mg/ metre^2 per day of prednisolone and this quickly and completely clears the proteinuria in most cases. This steroid dosage should be reduced and "tailed off" after four weeks as all uncomplicated cases will have remitted by this time.

5 - Relapse occurs in about half the number of patients, and these require longer individually tailored steroid therapy

4 - This steroid dose is gradually reduced and ceased after 4 weeks when uncomplicated cases will have remitted

3 - Prednisolone (60mg/ m^2/day) is the treatment of choice for "minimal change" disease in children and clears up proteinuria in most cases

8 - Checking for myeloid suppression by weekly blood counts

7 - Cyclophosphamide (3mg/kg) daily is 2nd-line treatment for non-responders to steroids

6 - Steroids, immunosuppressants and plasmapheresis are helpful in rapidly progressive glomerulonephritides, but many cases of nephrotic syndrome progress to chronic renal failure

Approximately half of all minimal change patients will never relapse again, but the other half do have relapses and will require longer, individually tailored, steroid therapy. In steroid non-responders, cyclophosphamide 3.0mg/Kg/day (as an immunosuppressant) is the next choice and is continued for at least eight weeks, checking for myelosuppression by weekly blood counts. The case for high dose steroids and immunosuppressants for treating nephrotic syndrome due to other histologies is not compelling and up to one third of patients with membranous glomerulonephritis will spontaneously remit – and a higher proportion of those with remediable underlying disease. When nephrotic syndrome accompanies the rapidly progressive glomerulonephritides, then steroids, immunosuppressants and plasmapheresis (as outlined above) may have a role to play. Unfortunately, many cases of nephrotic syndrome progress to chronic renal failure.

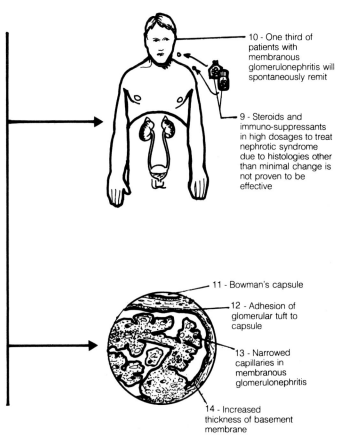

10 - One third of patients with membranous glomerulonephritis will spontaneously remit

9 - Steroids and immuno-suppressants in high dosages to treat nephrotic syndrome due to histologies other than minimal change is not proven to be effective

11 - Bowman's capsule

12 - Adhesion of glomerular tuft to capsule

13 - Narrowed capillaries in membranous glomerulonephritis

14 - Increased thickness of basement membrane

CHRONIC RENAL FAILURE (CRF)

Some 50 – 60% decrease in overall renal function (**GFR**) must occur before there is a significant effect on the blood chemistry (e.g. raised blood urea). Patients with the subclinical degree of renal impairment are said to have "diminished renal reserve". When the impairment becomes slightly more marked (e.g. **GFR**

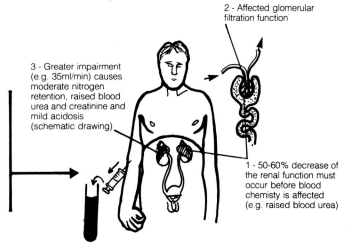

2 - Affected glomerular filtration function

3 - Greater impairment (e.g. 35ml/min) causes moderate nitrogen retention, raised blood urea and creatinine and mild acidosis (schematic drawing)

1 - 50-60% decrease of the renal function must occur before blood chemisty is affected (e.g. raised blood urea)

35ml/minute), there is moderate nitrogen retention (with raised blood urea and creatinine levels) and mild acidosis. At this stage nocturia and vague ill-health might be the first symptoms; hypertension, either as a cause or effect of the renal failure might be noted. The renal impairment may remain static at this level for a long time with the raised levels of nitrogen catabolites themselves creating an osmotic diuresis promoting their excretion by surviving nephrons, and thus finding an equilibrium plateau concentration in the blood. These patients have compensated renal insufficiency and manage without treatment out in the community, but are in danger of a sudden worsening of renal function during infections, losses of fluid and electrolytes (e.g. precipitated by diarrhoea and vomiting) or other stresses (e.g. major surgery). Further renal damage produces overt chronic renal failure (CRF) with significant nitrogen retention (uraemia), anaemia, deranged plasma electrolytes, acidosis, hypertension, neuromuscular and gastrointestinal symptoms and signs. Untreated, this often progresses and is fatal.

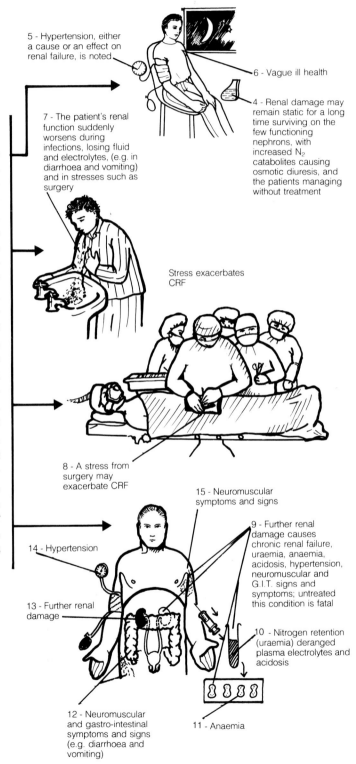

5 - Hypertension, either a cause or an effect on renal failure, is noted

6 - Vague ill health

4 - Renal damage may remain static for a long time surviving on the few functioning nephrons, with increased N_2 catabolites causing osmotic diuresis, and the patients managing without treatment

7 - The patient's renal function suddenly worsens during infections, losing fluid and electrolytes, (e.g. in diarrhoea and vomiting) and in stresses such as surgery

Stress exacerbates CRF

8 - A stress from surgery may exacerbate CRF

15 - Neuromuscular symptoms and signs

14 - Hypertension

9 - Further renal damage causes chronic renal failure, uraemia, anaemia, acidosis, hypertension, neuromuscular and G.I.T. signs and symptoms; untreated this condition is fatal

13 - Further renal damage

10 - Nitrogen retention (uraemia) deranged plasma electrolytes and acidosis

12 - Neuromuscular and gastro-intestinal symptoms and signs (e.g. diarrhoea and vomiting)

11 - Anaemia

Whilst the major causes of **CRF** vary from continent to continent and with age, the European data show that of the patients with CRF, 40% are caused by chronic glomerulonephritis, 20% by pyelonephritis (or more accurately: infection complicating existing renal disease, e.g. obstructive uropathy, interstitial nephritis, vesco-ureteric reflux etc), 10% by polycystic kidneys, 9% by diabetic nephrosclerosis, 7% by hypertensive vascular disease. It should be noted that chronic glomerulonephritis may follow a well-documented episode of acute glomerulonephritis or nephrotic syndrome – either immediately or after a latent period and the rate of progression varies enormously. Sometimes there may be no history of prior renal disease.

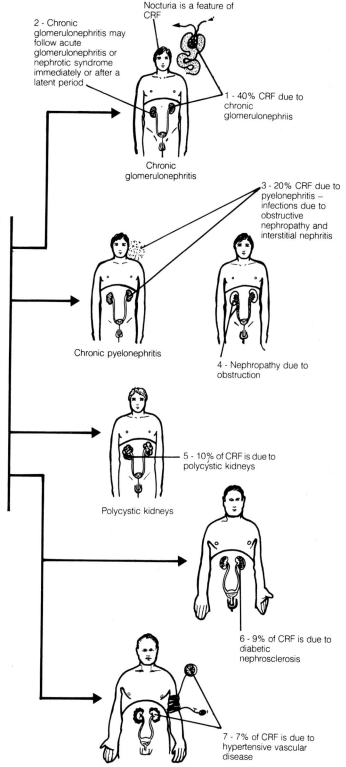

Nocturia is a feature of CRF

2 - Chronic glomerulonephritis may follow acute glomerulonephritis or nephrotic syndrome immediately or after a latent period

1 - 40% CRF due to chronic glomerulonephriis

Chronic glomerulonephritis

3 - 20% CRF due to pyelonephritis – infections due to obstructive nephropathy and interstitial nephritis

Chronic pyelonephritis

4 - Nephropathy due to obstruction

5 - 10% of CRF is due to polycystic kidneys

Polycystic kidneys

6 - 9% of CRF is due to diabetic nephrosclerosis

7 - 7% of CRF is due to hypertensive vascular disease

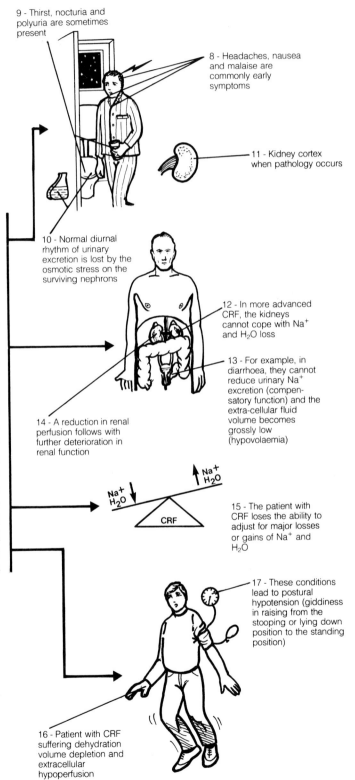

9 - Thirst, nocturia and polyuria are sometimes present

8 - Headaches, nausea and malaise are commonly early symptoms

11 - Kidney cortex when pathology occurs

10 - Normal diurnal rhythm of urinary excretion is lost by the osmotic stress on the surviving nephrons

12 - In more advanced CRF, the kidneys cannot cope with Na^+ and H_2O loss

13 - For example, in diarrhoea, they cannot reduce urinary Na^+ excretion (compensatory function) and the extra-cellular fluid volume becomes grossly low (hypovolaemia)

14 - A reduction in renal perfusion follows with further deterioration in renal function

Na^+ H_2O

Na^+ H_2O

CRF

15 - The patient with CRF loses the ability to adjust for major losses or gains of Na^+ and H_2O

17 - These conditions lead to postural hypotension (giddiness in raising from the stooping or lying down position to the standing position)

16 - Patient with CRF suffering dehydration volume depletion and extracellular hypoperfusion

Clinically, nausea, headaches and malaise or fatigue are common early symptoms, along with thirst, nocturia and sometimes polyuria. The normal diurnal rhythm of urinary excretion is lost by the osmotic stress on the surviving nephrons. Each surviving nephron is handling unusually large quantities of solutes and water and loses its concentrating and later diluting capacity – thus the urine in **CRF** has the same osmolality as plasma (isosthenuria). In more advanced **CRF**, the capacity of the kidneys to adjust to sudden changes in sodium and water loss becomes less efficient and, for example, an acute attack of diarrhoea cannot be accompanied by a compensatory reduction in the urinary sodium output; the extracellular fluid volume consequently becomes acutely contracted (hypovolaemia) with a reduction in renal perfusion and further deterioration in renal function occurs. Thus the patient

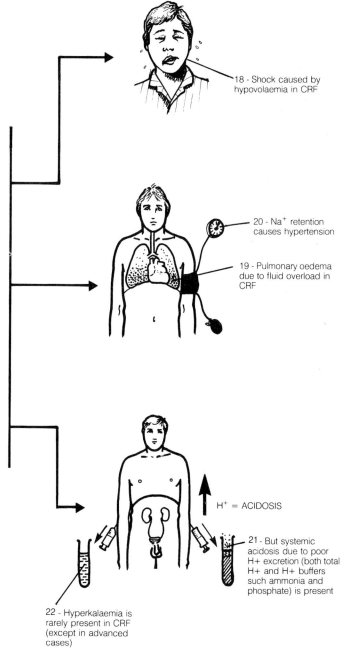

18 - Shock caused by hypovolaemia in CRF

20 - Na$^+$ retention causes hypertension

19 - Pulmonary oedema due to fluid overload in CRF

with **CRF** walks a "tight rope" facing the problems of dehydration, volume depletion and hypoperfusion on the one hand and fluid overload with pulmonary oedema on the other. However, assuming no such catastrophe occurs, a slow net retention of sodium is common in CRF and is a major contributor to the hypertension of CRF. Indeed, a normotensive patient with CRF usually has a sodium losing state, (commonly seen with polycystic disease and chronic urinary obstruction, and occasionally with phenacetin nephropathy and infection). Disturbed potassium balance is less common in **CRF** before the advanced stages, (when hyperkalaemia may become a dangerous complication), but a systemic acidosis is almost inevitably due to the direct deficit in total H$^+$ excretion and due to the reduced excretion of the H$^+$ buffers, (notably ammonia and phosphate).

H$^+$ = ACIDOSIS

21 - But systemic acidosis due to poor H+ excretion (both total H+ and H+ buffers such ammonia and phosphate) is present

22 - Hyperkalaemia is rarely present in CRF (except in advanced cases)

Calcium metabolism is disturbed in CRF for multiple reasons. In CRF, phosphate is retained and this tends to lower the blood calcium with an enhanced chance of metastatic/ectopic sites of calcification. The tendency to a lowering of the blood calcium causes secondary hyperparathyroidism which can cause the clinical, radiological and histological changes of osteitis fibrosa. Furthermore, there is a reduced renal production of 1,25 dihydroxycholecalciferol (1,25 **DHCC**) from 25 HCC and a refractoriness to the actions of vitamin D leading to the picture of osteomalacia, (called: renal osteomalacia) or rickets in children, and to reduced calcium absorption from the gut. The plasma calcium is usually in the low or low normal range in **CRF** and the composite picture of bone disease is termed renal osteodystrophy.

1 - In CRF calcium is lowered in blood because phosphorus is retained, resulting in calcification in ectopic sites

2 - Conjunctival calcification

3 - This low blood calcium causes secondary hyperparathyroidism resulting in bone resorption with cystic spaces or osteitis fibrosa

4 - Furthermore, there is reduced renal production of 1,25 DHCC from 25HCC resulting in a failure to utilize Vit. D with consequent renal osteomalacia or rickets in children

5 - Low blood calcium

12 - Bossing of forehead in rickets

11 - The plasma Ca is low in CRF and the disease termed "Renal Osteodystrophy"

6 - Clinical features of rickets

7 - Poor Ca absorption from gut

8 - Rickets, with weakness of bones, pain and fracture

9 - Thick cartilage and poor bone formation (renal osteomalacia)

10 - Bow legs

The rise in the blood urea with the reduction in GFR was blamed for the gastrointestinal, neuromuscular, cutaneous and haematological phenomena occurring in CRF as well as the late sequelae such as pericarditis.

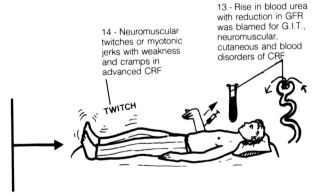

14 - Neuromuscular twitches or myotonic jerks with weakness and cramps in advanced CRF

13 - Rise in blood urea with reduction in GFR was blamed for G.I.T., neuromuscular, cutaneous and blood disorders of CRF

TWITCH

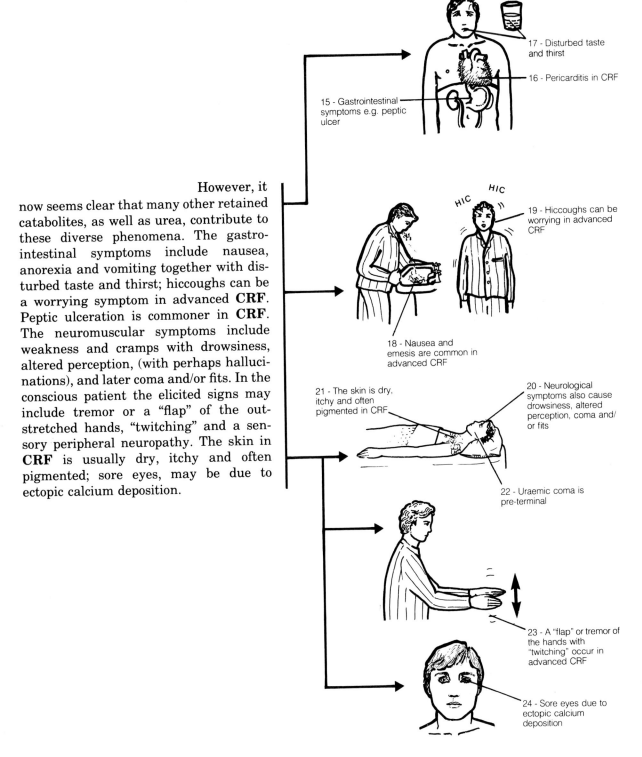

17 - Disturbed taste and thirst

16 - Pericarditis in CRF

15 - Gastrointestinal symptoms e.g. peptic ulcer

However, it now seems clear that many other retained catabolites, as well as urea, contribute to these diverse phenomena. The gastrointestinal symptoms include nausea, anorexia and vomiting together with disturbed taste and thirst; hiccoughs can be a worrying symptom in advanced **CRF**. Peptic ulceration is commoner in **CRF**. The neuromuscular symptoms include weakness and cramps with drowsiness, altered perception, (with perhaps hallucinations), and later coma and/or fits. In the conscious patient the elicited signs may include tremor or a "flap" of the outstretched hands, "twitching" and a sensory peripheral neuropathy. The skin in **CRF** is usually dry, itchy and often pigmented; sore eyes, may be due to ectopic calcium deposition.

HIC HIC

19 - Hiccoughs can be worrying in advanced CRF

18 - Nausea and emesis are common in advanced CRF

21 - The skin is dry, itchy and often pigmented in CRF

20 - Neurological symptoms also cause drowsiness, altered perception, coma and/ or fits

22 - Uraemic coma is pre-terminal

23 - A "flap" or tremor of the hands with "twitching" occur in advanced CRF

24 - Sore eyes due to ectopic calcium deposition

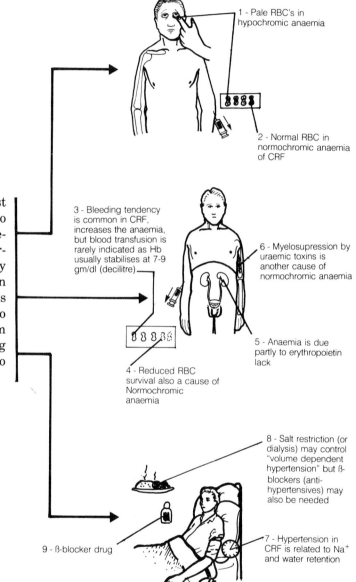

1 - Pale RBC's in hypochromic anaemia

2 - Normal RBC in normochromic anaemia of CRF

3 - Bleeding tendency is common in CRF, increases the anaemia, but blood transfusion is rarely indicated as Hb usually stabilises at 7-9 gm/dl (decilitre)

6 - Myelosupression by uraemic toxins is another cause of normochromic anaemia

5 - Anaemia is due partly to erythropoietin lack

4 - Reduced RBC survival also a cause of Normochromic anaemia

8 - Salt restriction (or dialysis) may control "volume dependent hypertension" but ß-blockers (anti-hypertensives) may also be needed

9 - ß-blocker drug

7 - Hypertension in CRF is related to Na^+ and water retention

A normochromic anaemia is almost universal in CRF, partially due to erythropoietin lack, partially due to reduced red cell survival and possibly partially due to direct myelosuppression by uraemic toxins. The haemoglobin often stabilises at 7-9g/dl and transfusion is reserved for specific indications, (as it also transfuses a nitrogen and potassium load). There is an increased bleeding tendency in CRF which may contribute to the anaemia.

Hypertension has been mentioned as being very common in advanced CRF and is usually related to the sodium and water retention. This "volume dependent hypertension" is usually controllable by salt restriction or dialysis. ß-blockers (the antihypertensive agents of first choice) may be needed also. Occasionally renin dependent hypertension occurs in CRF and prove difficult to control; rare patients on dialysis require bilateral nephrectomy to control this type of hypertension. Whatever the cause, hypertension demands prompt and effective treatment as it may exacerbate renal failure.

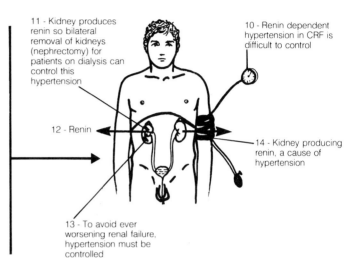

11 - Kidney produces renin so bilateral removal of kidneys (nephrectomy) for patients on dialysis can control this hypertension

10 - Renin dependent hypertension in CRF is difficult to control

12 - Renin

14 - Kidney producing renin, a cause of hypertension

13 - To avoid ever worsening renal failure, hypertension must be controlled

Management of CRF

The immediate questions that the clinician must seek to answer relate to the underlying cause of the renal failure, the degree of loss of renal function and the discovery of any reversible factors contributing to the decreased renal function, together with the correction of any life-threatening complications at presentation.

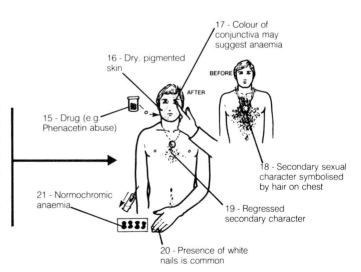

17 - Colour of conjunctiva may suggest anaemia

16 - Dry, pigmented skin

BEFORE

AFTER

15 - Drug (e.g. Phenacetin abuse)

18 - Secondary sexual character symbolised by hair on chest

21 - Normochromic anaemia

19 - Regressed secondary character

20 - Presence of white nails is common

The **history** may allow a **tentative diagnosis** (e.g phenacetin abuse) or at least give an idea concerning the "chronicity" of the CRF, (e.g. a long history of ill-health with nocturia for a year or more) and the examination may confirm the "chronic" features: dry, pigmented skin, anaemia, some regression of secondary sexual features, white nails etc. The **physical examination** may also assist in the diagnosis if the kidneys are palpable (e.g. polycystic disease, hydronephrosis). The blood pressure, presence of a pericardial friction rub, state of hydration and level or cerebration are also important clinical assessments.

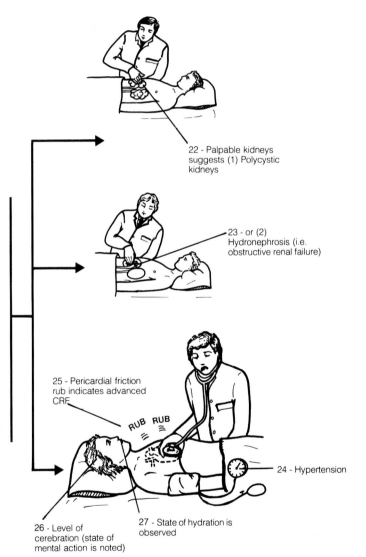

22 - Palpable kidneys suggests (1) Polycystic kidneys

23 - or (2) Hydronephrosis (i.e. obstructive renal failure)

25 - Pericardial friction rub indicates advanced CRF

RUB RUB

24 - Hypertension

26 - Level of cerebration (state of mental action is noted)

27 - State of hydration is observed

Measurement of the **blood electrolyte levels** and **urea** and **creatinine**, together with a 24 hour creatinine clearance (followed by a direct **GFR** measurement) provide a rapid screening for hyperkalaemia and overall renal function. Blood calcium, phosphate, magnesium, uric acid, glucose and hepatitis B antigen are also routinely monitored. **Renal tract imaging** is next performed after plain abdominal films have been examined (e.g. for calculi, nephrocalcinosis, T.B.). When deemed safe, modern high dose **IVU** with tomography is useful, particularly for diagnosing obstructive uropathy (often surgically correctable), and bilateral shrunken kidneys ("end-stage renal failure" – requiring no further diagnostic procedures as this diagnosis is quite irreversible). **Ultrasound** or **C.T.** scanning are alternative imaging procedures.

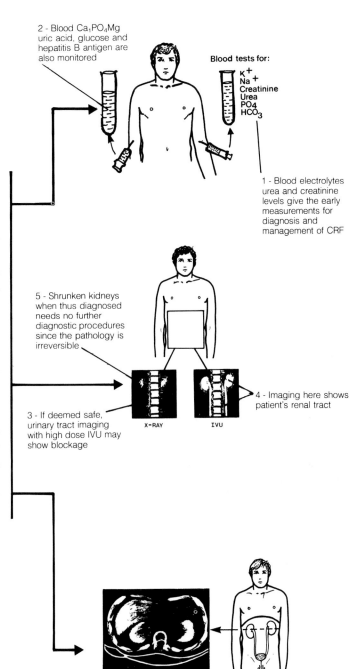

2 - Blood Ca_1PO_4Mg uric acid, glucose and hepatitis B antigen are also monitored

Blood tests for:
K^+
Na^+
Creatinine
Urea
PO_4
HCO_3

1 - Blood electrolytes urea and creatinine levels give the early measurements for diagnosis and management of CRF

5 - Shrunken kidneys when thus diagnosed needs no further diagnostic procedures since the pathology is irreversible

3 - If deemed safe, urinary tract imaging with high dose IVU may show blockage

X-RAY   IVU

4 - Imaging here shows patient's renal tract

C.T. Scan

6 - C.T. scan is an alternative imaging procedure

When the diagnosis is not clear, renal biopsy is indicated.

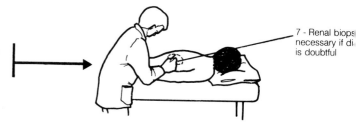

7 - Renal biops
necessary if di
is doubtful

The **reversible factors** to be searched for and treated in **CRF** are: i) Obstruction. ii) Infection. iii) Hypertension. iv) Fluid and electrolyte imbalance (both dehydration and overhydration). v) Hypercalcaemia.

Once correctable factors have been reversed, the overall renal function is reassessed by blood urea and creatinine levels, **GFR** and uraemic symptoms. The patients then divide into two groups: those for whom conservative management is appropriate and those requiring dialysis or transplantation.

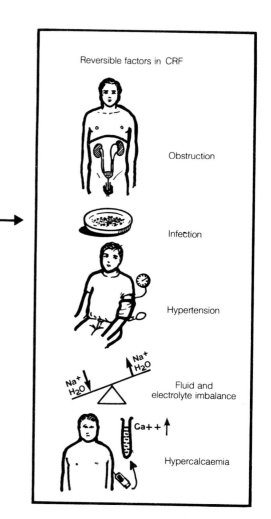

Reversible factors in CRF

Obstruction

Infection

Hypertension

Fluid and electrolyte imbalance

Hypercalcaemia

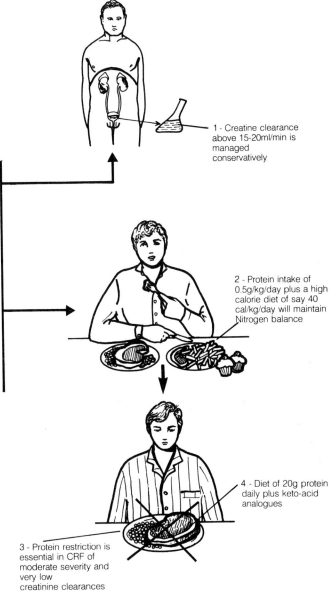

1 - Creatine clearance above 15-20ml/min is managed conservatively

Conservative Management of CRF –
For patients with a creatinine clearance of more that 15-20ml/min, conservative management is usually satisfactory. In order to maintain nitrogen balance over a long period, a protein intake of approximately 0.5g/Kg/day is needed together with a high calorie intake – at least 40 cal/Kg/day derived from fat and carbohydrate sources. However, temporarily, patients with very low creatinine clearances can be kept in nitrogen balance by further protein restriction, (diets containing 20g protein daily, plus keto-acid analogues).

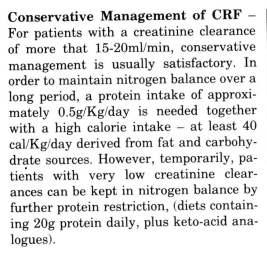

2 - Protein intake of 0.5g/kg/day plus a high calorie diet of say 40 cal/kg/day will maintain Nitrogen balance

4 - Diet of 20g protein daily plus keto-acid analogues

3 - Protein restriction is essential in CRF of moderate severity and very low creatinine clearances

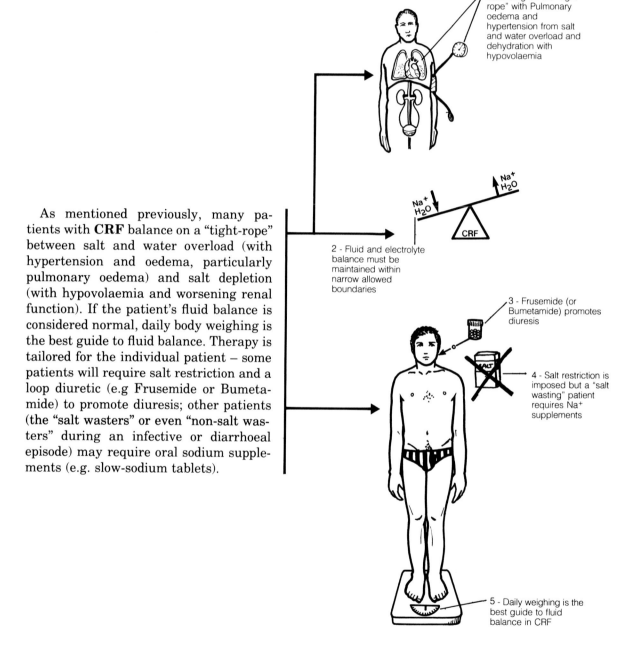

As mentioned previously, many patients with **CRF** balance on a "tight-rope" between salt and water overload (with hypertension and oedema, particularly pulmonary oedema) and salt depletion (with hypovolaemia and worsening renal function). If the patient's fluid balance is considered normal, daily body weighing is the best guide to fluid balance. Therapy is tailored for the individual patient – some patients will require salt restriction and a loop diuretic (e.g Frusemide or Bumetamide) to promote diuresis; other patients (the "salt wasters" or even "non-salt wasters" during an infective or diarrhoeal episode) may require oral sodium supplements (e.g. slow-sodium tablets).

1 - Patient with CRF balancing on the "tight rope" with Pulmonary oedema and hypertension from salt and water overload and dehydration with hypovolaemia

2 - Fluid and electrolyte balance must be maintained within narrow allowed boundaries

3 - Frusemide (or Bumetamide) promotes diuresis

4 - Salt restriction is imposed but a "salt wasting" patient requires Na^+ supplements

5 - Daily weighing is the best guide to fluid balance in CRF

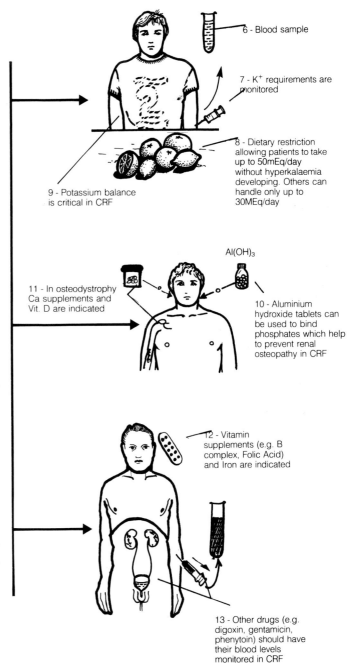

6 - Blood sample

7 - K⁺ requirements are monitored

8 - Dietary restriction allowing patients to take up to 50mEq/day without hyperkalaemia developing. Others can handle only up to 30MEq/day

9 - Potassium balance is critical in CRF

Potassium requirements are also monitored and there is a dietary restriction. Most patients will be able to consume up to 50mEq/day without becoming hyperkalaemic but others are unable to handle an intake of more than 30mEq/day and this is difficult to accommodate within the necessary diet.

Al(OH)₃

11 - In osteodystrophy Ca supplements and Vit. D are indicated

10 - Aluminium hydroxide tablets can be used to bind phosphates which help to prevent renal osteopathy in CRF

A strong case can be made for commencing phosphate binding agents (e.g. aluminium hydroxide tablets) as prophylaxis against renal osteodystrophy early in the course of **CRF**, (e.g creatinine clearance less than 50ml/min) – Occasionally, with advancing osteodystrophy, calcium supplements and vitamin D analogues are indicated.

12 - Vitamin supplements (e.g. B complex, Folic Acid) and Iron are indicated

Vitamin supplements (especially vitamin B complex, Folic acid and Iron) are indicated. Other drug prescriptions are only made after very careful consideration of the mode of drug elimination and often with monitoring of drug levels (e.g. digoxin, gentamicin, phenytoin).

13 - Other drugs (e.g. digoxin, gentamicin, phenytoin) should have their blood levels monitored in CRF

Dialysis/Transplantion for CRF

Patients with severe **CRF** should be referred early to a specialist nephrology centre for assessment of suitability for a dialysis or transplantation programme which they will require when the **GFR** falls to approximately 10% of the normal. The accepted indication for dialysis (or transplant) include the chronic malaise that accompanies advanced **CRF** (e.g. when the serum creatinine is 1000-2000μmol/Litre) and other specific indications include: Hyperkalaemia, pericarditis, neurological complication (clouding of consciousness, fits, flaps, neuropathy) and control of fluid overload (particularly pulmonary oedema).

Detailed description of dialysis or the results of renal transplantation are beyond the scope of this chapter but it should be realised that both are attended by complications and neither return patients to a normal life expectancy. In the absence of certain well established contraindications, transplantation of a kidney from a histocompatible living donor relative is the most successful therapy in adults, (excepting the elderly).

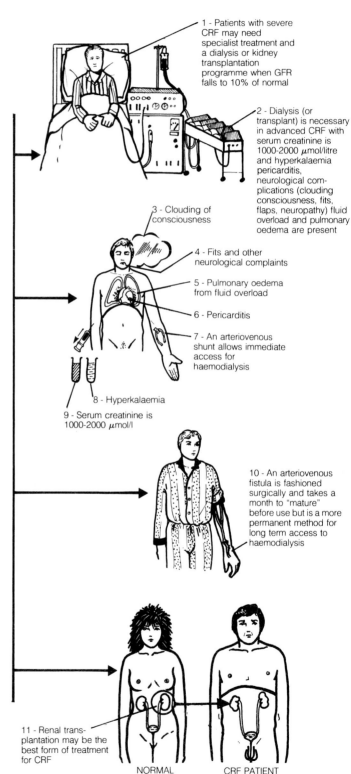

1 - Patients with severe CRF may need specialist treatment and a dialysis or kidney transplantation programme when GFR falls to 10% of normal

2 - Dialysis (or transplant) is necessary in advanced CRF with serum creatinine is 1000-2000 μmol/litre and hyperkalaemia pericarditis, neurological complications (clouding consciousness, fits, flaps, neuropathy) fluid overload and pulmonary oedema are present

3 - Clouding of consciousness

4 - Fits and other neurological complaints

5 - Pulmonary oedema from fluid overload

6 - Pericarditis

7 - An arteriovenous shunt allows immediate access for haemodialysis

8 - Hyperkalaemia

9 - Serum creatinine is 1000-2000 μmol/l

10 - An arteriovenous fistula is fashioned surgically and takes a month to "mature" before use but is a more permanent method for long term access to haemodialysis

11 - Renal transplantation may be the best form of treatment for CRF

NORMAL   CRF PATIENT

OBSTRUCTIVE UROPATHY

Obstructive uropathy may present with renal colic (due to calculi), with the more chronic loin ache of hydronephrosis or with post-renal failure.

The common causes are:–
  i) Tumours – Genito-urinary tract tumours
  – Retroperitoneal tumours (e.g. lymphomas)
  – Pelvic tumours (e.g. carcinoma of cervix).

  ii) Renal Calculi

  iii) Prostatic enlargement

  iv) Retroperitoneal fibrosis.

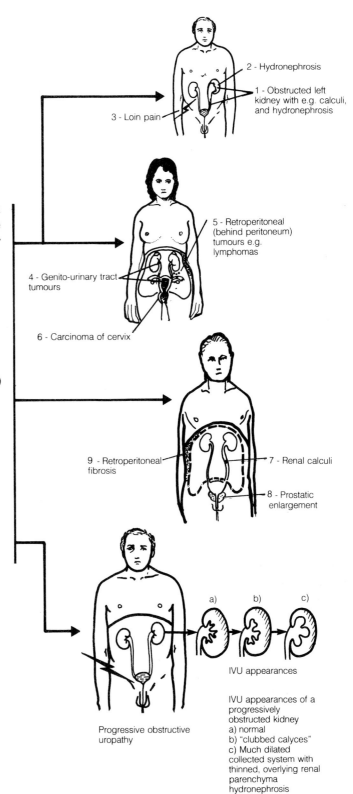

2 - Hydronephrosis

1 - Obstructed left kidney with e.g. calculi, and hydronephrosis

3 - Loin pain

5 - Retroperitoneal (behind peritoneum) tumours e.g. lymphomas

4 - Genito-urinary tract tumours

6 - Carcinoma of cervix

9 - Retroperitoneal fibrosis

7 - Renal calculi

8 - Prostatic enlargement

a) b) c)

IVU appearances

IVU appearances of a progressively obstructed kidney
a) normal
b) "clubbed calyces"
c) Much dilated collected system with thinned, overlying renal parenchyma hydronephrosis

Progressive obstructive uropathy

Genito-urinary Tract Tumours

The **management** of genito-urinary tumours is important. Wilms' tumour is a malignancy of young children, presenting usually as an abdominal mass and highly curable with surgery and modern radiotherapy with chemotherapy. Renal cell carcinoma, (hypernephroma, Grawitz cell tumour), is the commonest adult solid kidney tumour in adults tending to present late or with metastases; early nephrectomy may be curative but metastatic disease augurs poorly. Transitional cell carcinoma may arise from the renal pelvis, ureters or most commonly in the bladder and it may present with haematuria or obstructive uropathy. Early papillary growths are best resected at cystoscopy; more advanced growths are curable in approximately 40% of cases by skillful radiotherapy with or without cystectomy. Follow-up of patients following radiotherapy includes periodic cystoscopies as "salvage cystectomy" has proved curative in some late relapses.

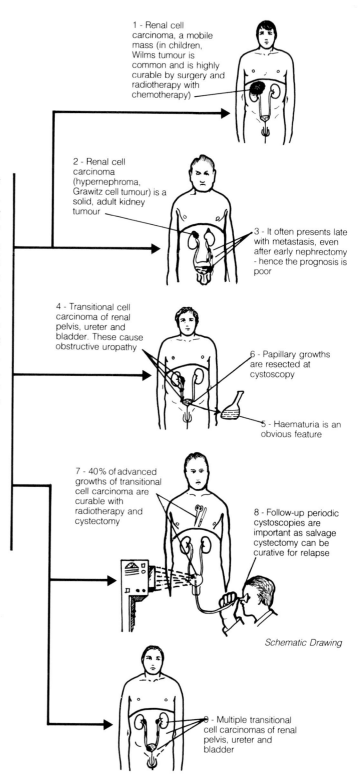

1 - Renal cell carcinoma, a mobile mass (in children, Wilms tumour is common and is highly curable by surgery and radiotherapy with chemotherapy)

2 - Renal cell carcinoma (hypernephroma, Grawitz cell tumour) is a solid, adult kidney tumour

3 - It often presents late with metastasis, even after early nephrectomy - hence the prognosis is poor

4 - Transitional cell carcinoma of renal pelvis, ureter and bladder. These cause obstructive uropathy

6 - Papillary growths are resected at cystoscopy

5 - Haematuria is an obvious feature

7 - 40% of advanced growths of transitional cell carcinoma are curable with radiotherapy and cystectomy

8 - Follow-up periodic cystoscopies are important as salvage cystectomy can be curative for relapse

Schematic Drawing

9 - Multiple transitional cell carcinomas of renal pelvis, ureter and bladder

Renal Calculi

G.U. tract calculi may cause obstructive uropathy, (with severe renal colic if the blockage is acute), with post-renal failure, or haemorrhage or infection. There are certain well-recognised predisposing factors in the causation of calculi – infection with urinary stasis, diverticula with stasis, hypercalcaemia due to any cause (e.g. hyperparathyroidism), hyperuricaemia, hyperoxaluria. However, the majority of the common mixed oxalate and phosphate stones/calculi are usually of obscure origin, (but the clinician should nevertheless search for an underlying and treatable predisposing cause). Unlike the mixed calculi, uric acid stones are not radio-opaque on the plain abdominal X-ray.

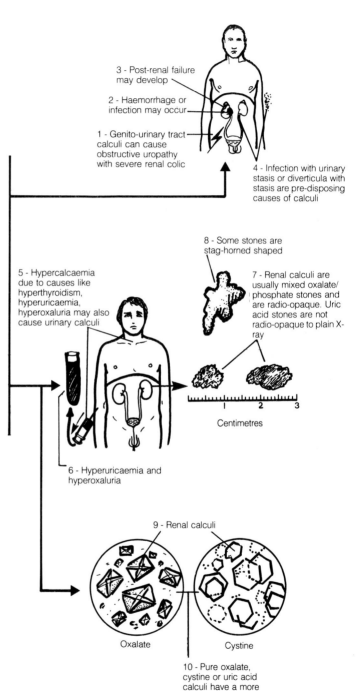

3 - Post-renal failure may develop

2 - Haemorrhage or infection may occur

1 - Genito-urinary tract calculi can cause obstructive uropathy with severe renal colic

4 - Infection with urinary stasis or diverticula with stasis are pre-disposing causes of calculi

8 - Some stones are stag-horned shaped

7 - Renal calculi are usually mixed oxalate/ phosphate stones and are radio-opaque. Uric acid stones are not radio-opaque to plain X-ray

5 - Hypercalcaemia due to causes like hyperthyroidism, hyperuricaemia, hyperoxaluria may also cause urinary calculi

Centimetres

6 - Hyperuricaemia and hyperoxaluria

9 - Renal calculi

Oxalate

Cystine

10 - Pure oxalate, cystine or uric acid calculi have a more regular crystalline appearance

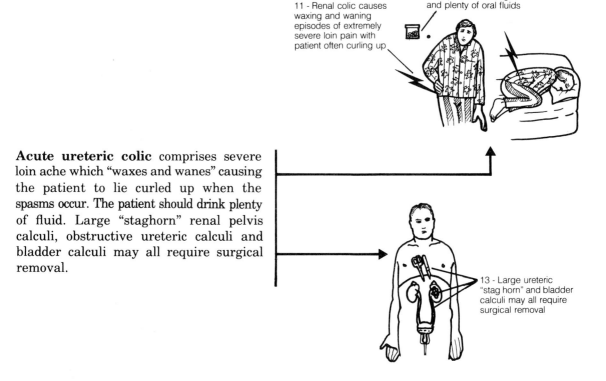

11 - Renal colic causes waxing and waning episodes of extremely severe loin pain with patient often curling up

12 - Treatment is by opiate analgesics and anti-spasmodic drugs and plenty of oral fluids

13 - Large ureteric "stag horn" and bladder calculi may all require surgical removal

Acute ureteric colic comprises severe loin ache which "waxes and wanes" causing the patient to lie curled up when the spasms occur. The patient should drink plenty of fluid. Large "staghorn" renal pelvis calculi, obstructive ureteric calculi and bladder calculi may all require surgical removal.

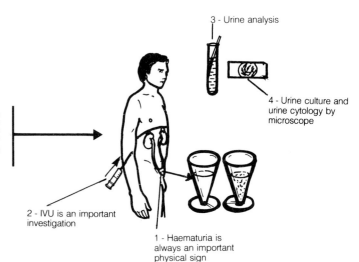

3 - Urine analysis

4 - Urine culture and urine cytology by microscope

2 - IVU is an important investigation

1 - Haematuria is always an important physical sign

Haematuria

Haematuria is a complaint demanding investigation in all patients (including IVU, urine analysis, urine cytology, urine culture and probably cystoscopy).

Whilst trauma is one cause, tumours and calculi in the GU tract must always be suspected as well as infections — (e.g. schistosomiasis, T.B.).

Occasionally, recurrent haematuria in children is due to a particular form of glomerulonephritis, diagnosable only on renal biopsy. Rarely, haematuria may be the presenting symptom of a bleeding diathesis. (i.e. a predisposition to diseases which cause bleeding).

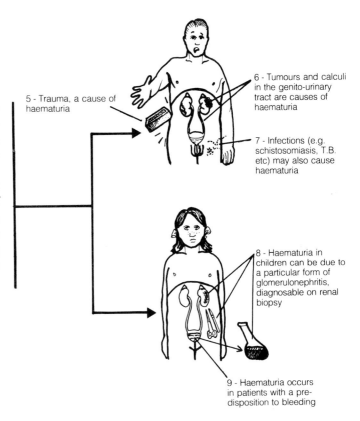

5 - Trauma, a cause of haematuria

6 - Tumours and calculi in the genito-urinary tract are causes of haematuria

7 - Infections (e.g. schistosomiasis, T.B. etc) may also cause haematuria

8 - Haematuria in children can be due to a particular form of glomerulonephritis, diagnosable on renal biopsy

9 - Haematuria occurs in patients with a pre-disposition to bleeding

Retroperitoneal Fibrosis

This rare condition, which may lead to obstructive uropathy is usually idiopathic or drug-related (e.g. methysergide). A progressive fibrosis of the retroperitoneal tissues of the posterior abdominal walls occurs obstructing one and then both ureters; later the inferior vena cava may be involved. Steroids are not very effective at preventing the progression but are worth a trial before relieving or diversionary surgery is employed.

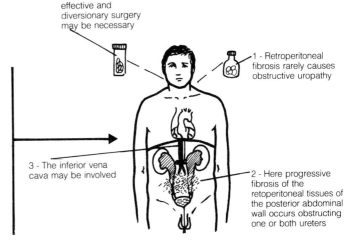

4 - Steroids are seldom effective and diversionary surgery may be necessary

1 - Retroperitoneal fibrosis rarely causes obstructive uropathy

3 - The inferior vena cava may be involved

2 - Here progressive fibrosis of the retoperitoneal tissues of the posterior abdominal wall occurs obstructing one or both ureters

Renal Artery Stenosis

This vascular disease is now recognised as an important, albeit rare, reversible cause of hypertension. In the elderly, it is usually caused by atherosclerosis whereas in younger age groups renal arterial wall "fibromuscular hyperplasia" is the cause.

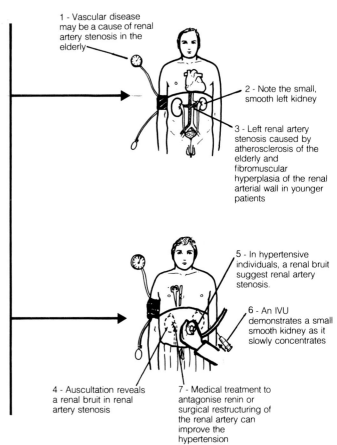

1 - Vascular disease may be a cause of renal artery stenosis in the elderly

2 - Note the small, smooth left kidney

3 - Left renal artery stenosis caused by atherosclerosis of the elderly and fibromuscular hyperplasia of the renal arterial wall in younger patients

In a typical case. a hypertensive individual is found to have a renal "bruit" and the IVU demonstrates a small smooth kidney on that side, the nephrogram appearing late and then showing increased enhancement as it concentrates the contrast material. If the renal artery stenosis is the cause of the hypertension then the serum renin will be high and therapy may be medical, (aimed at lowering or antagonising renin mediated hypertension), or surgical, (aimed at reconstructing the renal artery).

5 - In hypertensive individuals, a renal bruit suggest renal artery stenosis.

6 - An IVU demonstrates a small smooth kidney as it slowly concentrates

4 - Auscultation reveals a renal bruit in renal artery stenosis

7 - Medical treatment to antagonise renin or surgical restructuring of the renal artery can improve the hypertension

Renal Vein Thrombosis

This serious condition may lead to acute renal failure or, with a more slowly developing thrombosis, a nephrotic syndrome occurs.

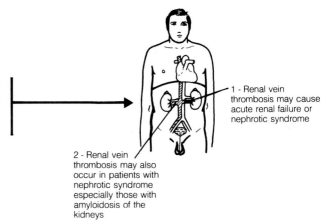

1 - Renal vein thrombosis may cause acute renal failure or nephrotic syndrome

2 - Renal vein thrombosis may also occur in patients with nephrotic syndrome especially those with amyloidosis of the kidneys

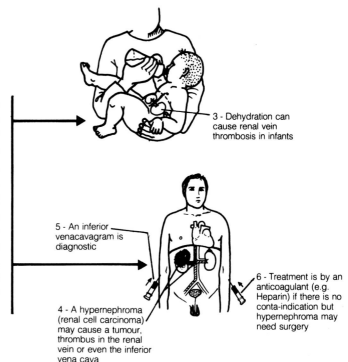

Renal vein thrombosis is more likely to occur in patients with the nephrotic syndrome of any aetiology, but particularly in patients with amyloidosis of the kidneys. In infants, severe dehydration is a well-recognised cause of renal vein thrombosis. A hypernephroma invading the renal venules and veins may form an obstructing tumour thrombus. An inferior venacavagram is the diagnostic test and anti-coagulation the treatment, (assuming no contra-indications) unless due to hypernephroma – when surgery may be indicated.

3 - Dehydration can cause renal vein thrombosis in infants

5 - An inferior venacavagram is diagnostic

6 - Treatment is by an anticoagulant (e.g. Heparin) if there is no conta-indication but hypernephroma may need surgery

4 - A hypernephroma (renal cell carcinoma) may cause a tumour, thrombus in the renal vein or even the inferior vena cava

URINARY TRACT INFECTIONS

Urinary tract infections (UTI) are very common, particularly in women (and especially during pregnancy). The majority of UTI present with symptoms of dysuria and frequency due to a cystitis; they are diagnosed by the finding of more than 10^5 organisms per ml. of "clean catch", mid-stream urine (MSU) and a raised white cell count in the urine. Culture allows identification, (usually a Gram negative aerobic bacillus and most commonly E.Coli). **Treatment** is with the appropriate antibiotic and adequate fluid intake, and it is the clinician's responsibility to check that the infection has been eradicated by a further MSU after cessation of antibiotic therapy.

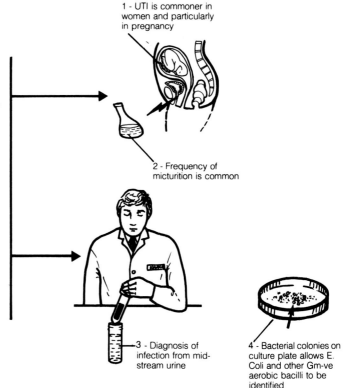

1 - UTI is commoner in women and particularly in pregnancy

2 - Frequency of micturition is common

3 - Diagnosis of infection from mid-stream urine

4 - Bacterial colonies on culture plate allows E. Coli and other Gm-ve aerobic bacilli to be identified

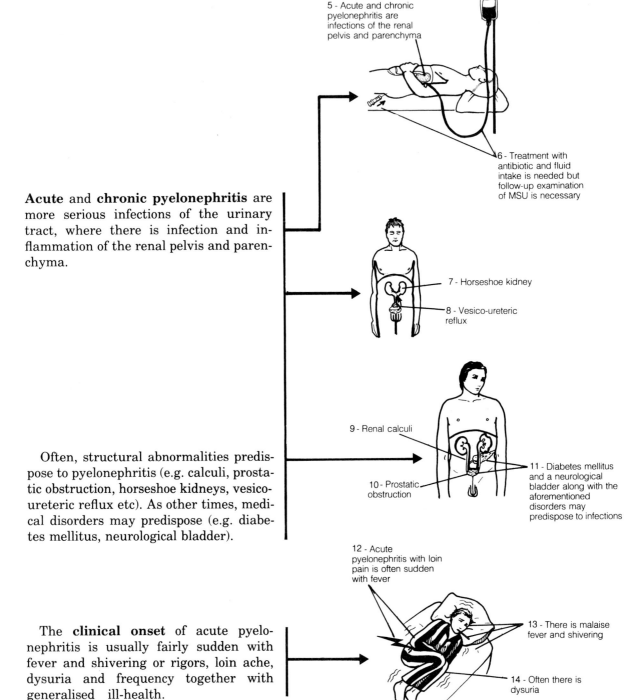

5 - Acute and chronic pyelonephritis are infections of the renal pelvis and parenchyma

6 - Treatment with antibiotic and fluid intake is needed but follow-up examination of MSU is necessary

7 - Horseshoe kidney

8 - Vesico-ureteric reflux

9 - Renal calculi

10 - Prostatic obstruction

11 - Diabetes mellitus and a neurological bladder along with the aforementioned disorders may predispose to infections

12 - Acute pyelonephritis with loin pain is often sudden with fever

13 - There is malaise fever and shivering

14 - Often there is dysuria

Acute and **chronic pyelonephritis** are more serious infections of the urinary tract, where there is infection and inflammation of the renal pelvis and parenchyma.

Often, structural abnormalities predispose to pyelonephritis (e.g. calculi, prostatic obstruction, horseshoe kidneys, vesicoureteric reflux etc). As other times, medical disorders may predispose (e.g. diabetes mellitus, neurological bladder).

The **clinical onset** of acute pyelonephritis is usually fairly sudden with fever and shivering or rigors, loin ache, dysuria and frequency together with generalised ill-health.

The loins are usually tender, investigations show a neutrophil leucocytosis and pyuria. The majority of first attacks of acute pyelonephritis are due to **E. coli** and other common infecting organisms are: **Proteus mirabilis, Klebsiella aerogenes, Streptococcus faecalis, Staphyloccus aureus.**

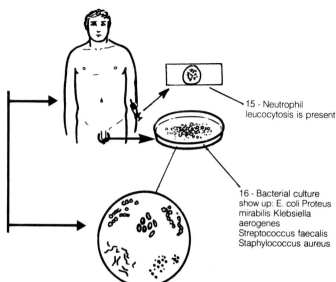

15 - Neutrophil leucocytosis is present

16 - Bacterial culture show up: E. coli Proteus mirabilis Klebsiella aerogenes Streptococcus faecalis Staphylococcus aureus

Chronic pyelonephritis with severe renal damage and CRF almost always occurs in kidneys with existing structural abnormalities – or kidneys damaged in childhood. Chronic pyelonephritis may then, after multiple pyelonephritis attacks, lead to small, shrunken contracted kidneys with coarse cortical scarring on **IVU**, (perhaps together with clubbed calyces). Other organisms, more commonly found in chronic rather than acute pyelonephritis, (and more commonly in a hospital patient population), are Proteus vulgaris and Pseudomonas pyocyanea. The **antibiotic treatment** of chronic pyelonephritis may need to be prolonged.

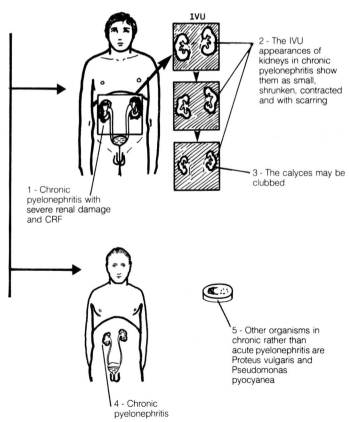

IVU

2 - The IVU appearances of kidneys in chronic pyelonephritis show them as small, shrunken, contracted and with scarring

3 - The calyces may be clubbed

1 - Chronic pyelonephritis with severe renal damage and CRF

5 - Other organisms in chronic rather than acute pyelonephritis are Proteus vulgaris and Pseudomonas pyocyanea

4 - Chronic pyelonephritis

Genito-urinary tract T.B. may cause pyuria with "no growth" on orthodox culture media; an early morning urine specimen cultured for some weeks on Lowenstein-Jensen medium is required for the diagnosis. G.U.–T.B. must never be forgotten as a cause of urinary tract infection.

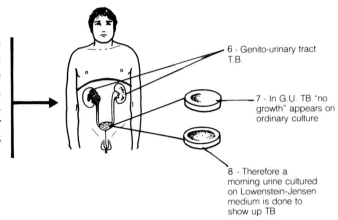

6 - Genito-urinary tract T.B.

7 - In G.U. TB "no growth" appears on ordinary culture

8 - Therefore a morning urine cultured on Lowenstein-Jensen medium is done to show up TB

RENAL PAPILLARY NECROSIS

Acute necrosis may occur as a complication of acute or chronic pyelonephritis. Other recognised predisposing illnesses include: diabetes mellitus, sickle cell anaemia, phenacetin abuse, obstructive uropathy and **T.B.** The necrosis is thought to be due to ischaemia in all these conditions. The patient may present with renal colic due to the painful passage of the shed papillae down the ureter or even with **ARF**. The **IVU** may be diagnostic.

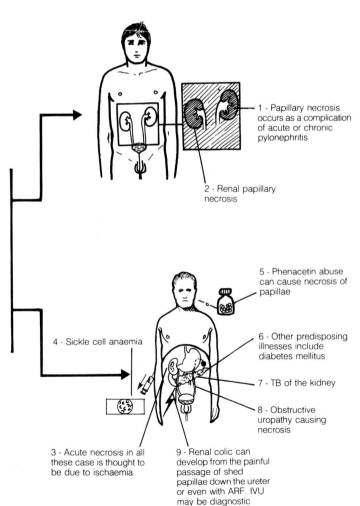

1 - Papillary necrosis occurs as a complication of acute or chronic pylonephritis

2 - Renal papillary necrosis

5 - Phenacetin abuse can cause necrosis of papillae

6 - Other predisposing illnesses include diabetes mellitus

7 - TB of the kidney

8 - Obstructive uropathy causing necrosis

4 - Sickle cell anaemia

3 - Acute necrosis in all these case is thought to be due to ischaemia

9 - Renal colic can develop from the painful passage of shed papillae down the ureter or even with ARF. IVU may be diagnostic

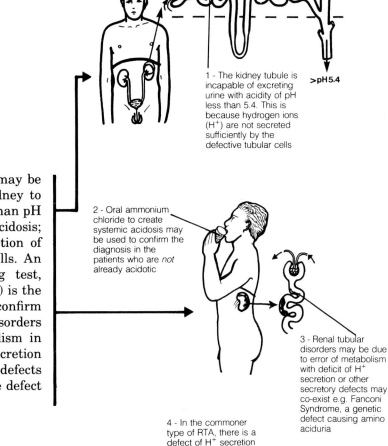

1 - The kidney tubule is incapable of excreting urine with acidity of pH less than 5.4. This is because hydrogen ions (H$^+$) are not secreted sufficiently by the defective tubular cells

>pH 5.4

RENAL TUBULAR ACIDOSIS

Renal Tubular Acidosis (**RTA**) may be defined as the inability of the kidney to excrete urine more acid, (lower), than pH 5.4 despite a systemic metabolic acidosis; its cause is a defect in the secretion of hydrogen ions (H$^+$) by tubular cells. An oral ammonium chloride loading test, (used to create a systemic acidosis) is the diagnostic test used to clinically confirm the diagnosis. Renal tubular disorders may be inborn errors of metabolism in which the tubular deficit in H$^+$ secretion is only one of several secreting defects (e.g. **Fanconi's syndrome**) or the defect may be single.

2 - Oral ammonium chloride to create systemic acidosis may be used to confirm the diagnosis in the patients who are *not* already acidotic

3 - Renal tubular disorders may be due to error of metabolism with deficit of H$^+$ secretion or other secretory defects may co-exist e.g. Fanconi Syndrome, a genetic defect causing amino aciduria

4 - In the commoner type of RTA, there is a defect of H$^+$ secretion into the distal collecting tubule. This defect is inherited or due to obstructive uropathy, pyelonephritis or hypercalcaemia

H$^+$

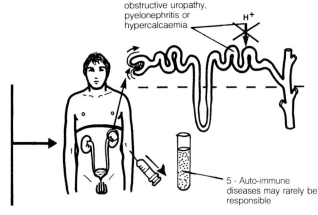

In the commoner form of renal tubular acidosis there is a single defect in the generation of a pH gradient by the distal tubule; this condition may be inherited or occur following obstructive uropathy, pyelonephritis or hypercalcaemia; cases have been reported following auto-immune diseases.

5 - Auto-immune diseases may rarely be responsible

Treatment consists of oral alkali (e.g. sodium bicarbonate tablets 3-10g (day) and oral potassium supplements will be needed by some patients; the prognosis of this type of **RTA** is good.

Proximal tubular RTA is a more serious condition that is less amenable to alkali therapy. The **PCT** is unable to secrete H^+ normally and so a substantial fraction of bicarbonate filtered by the glomerulus, (whose reabsorption depends on H^+ secretion), appears in the urine. There is a persistent and often severe hyperchloraemic acidosis that is resistant to treatment with alkalis. Rickets (osteomalacia) and potassium depletion are well recognised complications. Nephrocalcinosis (fine, renal medullary spiculation with calcium on X-ray – becoming more gross with time) is also a feature of **RTA** and may cause impairment of overall renal function. (This radiological appearance of nephrocalcinosis may also appear with chronic hypercalcaemia and in medullary sponge kidney).

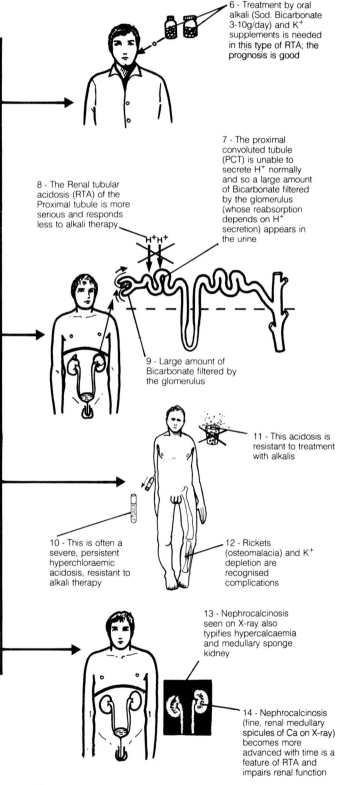

6 - Treatment by oral alkali (Sod. Bicarbonate 3-10g/day) and K^+ supplements is needed in this type of RTA; the prognosis is good

7 - The proximal convoluted tubule (PCT) is unable to secrete H^+ normally and so a large amount of Bicarbonate filtered by the glomerulus (whose reabsorption depends on H^+ secretion) appears in the urine

8 - The Renal tubular acidosis (RTA) of the Proximal tubule is more serious and responds less to alkali therapy

$H^+ H^+$

9 - Large amount of Bicarbonate filtered by the glomerulus

11 - This acidosis is resistant to treatment with alkalis

10 - This is often a severe, persistent hyperchloraemic acidosis, resistant to alkali therapy

12 - Rickets (osteomalacia) and K^+ depletion are recognised complications

13 - Nephrocalcinosis seen on X-ray also typifies hypercalcaemia and medullary sponge kidney

14 - Nephrocalcinosis (fine, renal medullary spicules of Ca on X-ray) becomes more advanced with time is a feature of RTA and impairs renal function

Fluid and Electrolyte Pathophysiology

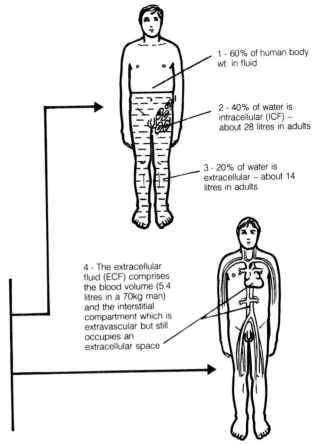

1 - 60% of human body wt. in fluid

2 - 40% of water is intracellular (ICF) – about 28 litres in adults

3 - 20% of water is extracellular – about 14 litres in adults

4 - The extracellular fluid (ECF) comprises the blood volume (5.4 litres in a 70kg man) and the interstitial compartment which is extravascular but still occupies an extracellular space

DISTURBANCES OF ELECTROLYTES

Approximately 60% of the human body weight is due to fluid, 40% being in the intracellular compartment, **ICF**, (approximately 28 litres in adults) and 20% in the extracellular compartment, (approximately 14 litres in adults). The extracellular fluid (**ECF**), comprises the blood volume (5.4 litres in 70Kg man) and the interstitial compartment, (that extravascular yet still extracellular space).

The distribution of electrolytes differs greatly between the **ECF** and **ICF** due to cell membrane transport mechanisms:

	ECF	ICF
Na^+	140mmol/l	12mmol/l
K^+	4	155
Cl^-	100	10
HCO_3^-	28	10
Mg^{++}	1	28
PO_4^{---}	1	105

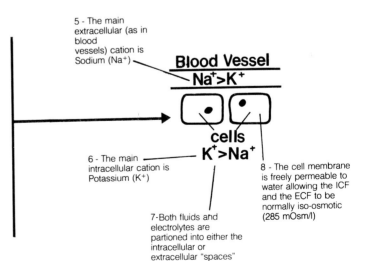

5 - The main extracellular (as in blood vessels) cation is Sodium (Na^+)

6 - The main intracellular cation is Potassium (K^+)

7 - Both fluids and electrolytes are partioned into either the intracellular or extracellular "spaces"

8 - The cell membrane is freely permeable to water allowing the ICF and the ECF to be normally iso-osmotic (285 mOsm/l)

Blood Vessel
$Na^+ > K^+$

cells
$K^+ > Na^+$

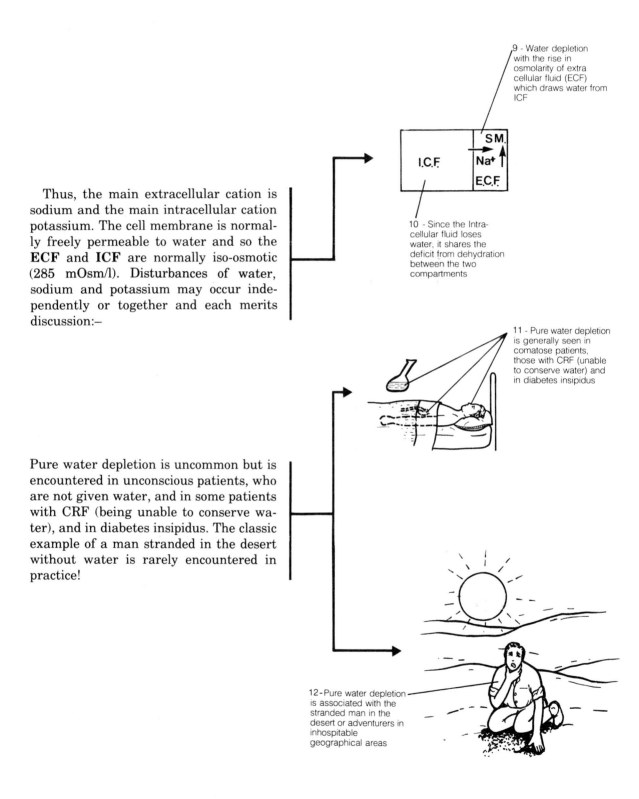

9 - Water depletion with the rise in osmolarity of extra cellular fluid (ECF) which draws water from ICF

Thus, the main extracellular cation is sodium and the main intracellular cation potassium. The cell membrane is normally freely permeable to water and so the **ECF** and **ICF** are normally iso-osmotic (285 mOsm/l). Disturbances of water, sodium and potassium may occur independently or together and each merits discussion:–

10 - Since the Intracellular fluid loses water, it shares the deficit from dehydration between the two compartments

11 - Pure water depletion is generally seen in comatose patients, those with CRF (unable to conserve water) and in diabetes insipidus

Pure water depletion is uncommon but is encountered in unconscious patients, who are not given water, and in some patients with CRF (being unable to conserve water), and in diabetes insipidus. The classic example of a man stranded in the desert without water is rarely encountered in practice!

12 - Pure water depletion is associated with the stranded man in the desert or adventurers in inhospitable geographical areas

64

The physiology of pure water depletion begins with a rise in the osmolarity of **ECF** which draws water from the **ICF** – sharing the deficit between the two compartments. The serum sodium rises and, if renal function is normal, a small volume of concentrated urine is passed. The increase in osmotic pressure leads to thirst, drowsiness and later coma. When the depletion is severe, the reduction in body fluids leads to oliguria and pre-renal failure. **Treatment** is by oral water or intravenous 5% dextrose.

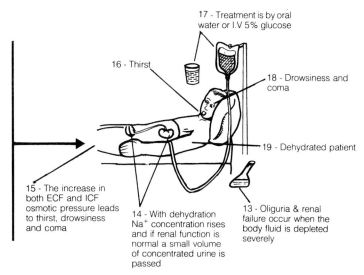

17 - Treatment is by oral water or I.V 5% glucose

16 - Thirst

18 - Drowsiness and coma

19 - Dehydrated patient

15 - The increase in both ECF and ICF osmotic pressure leads to thirst, drowsiness and coma

14 - With dehydration Na$^+$ concentration rises and if renal function is normal a small volume of concentrated urine is passed

13 - Oliguria & renal failure occur when the body fluid is depleted severely

More common is combined salt and water depletion that is commonly seen with fluid loss from the gastrointestinal tract, (diarrhoea, vomiting, fistula), or urinary tract (Addison's disease, diabetes mellitus). The **ECF** osmotic pressure tends to fall or remain normal as there is no rise in the serum sodium and thus the volume depletion is not shared with the **ICF**. Clinically, this produces the picture of hypovolaemia with peripheral vasoconstriction (pale and cold extremities) and rapid, thin pulse with low blood pressure.

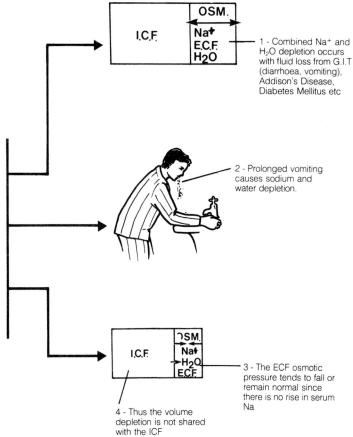

I.C.F. OSM. Na$^+$ E.C.F. H$_2$O

1 - Combined Na$^+$ and H$_2$O depletion occurs with fluid loss from G.I.T (diarrhoea, vomiting), Addison's Disease, Diabetes Mellitus etc

2 - Prolonged vomiting causes sodium and water depletion.

I.C.F. OSM. Na$^+$ H$_2$O ECF.

3 - The ECF osmotic pressure tends to fall or remain normal since there is no rise in serum Na

4 - Thus the volume depletion is not shared with the ICF

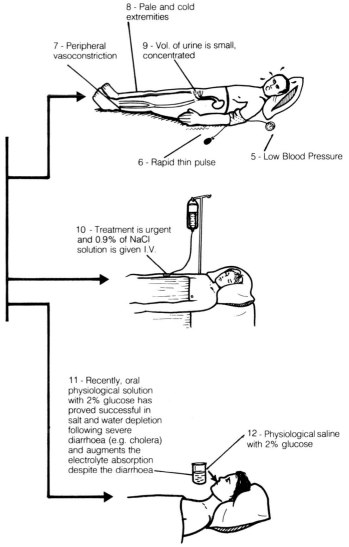

8 - Pale and cold extremities

7 - Peripheral vasoconstriction

9 - Vol. of urine is small, concentrated

6 - Rapid thin pulse

5 - Low Blood Pressure

The urine is usually small in volume and concentrated. The **Treatment** is with 0.9% sodium chloride solution (physiological saline) intravenously. Of great interest and importance in recent years has been the observation that severe salt and water depletion that occurs following severe diarrhoea, (as in cholera), can often be replaced by **oral** administration of physiological saline supplemented with 2% glucose, which augments the electrolyte absorption, despite the diarrhoea.

10 - Treatment is urgent and 0.9% of NaCl solution is given I.V.

11 - Recently, oral physiological solution with 2% glucose has proved successful in salt and water depletion following severe diarrhoea (e.g. cholera) and augments the electrolyte absorption despite the diarrhoea

12 - Physiological saline with 2% glucose

13 - Head trauma may lead to excessive ADH secretion

Water intoxication is unusual but may occur in renal disease or due to inappropriate secretion of **ADH** (e.g. following head injury or ectopically by a tumour, notably small cell bronchial carcinoma). The excess water is distributed evenly throughout ECF and ICF, and plasma electrolytes and osmolality are low. The urine tends to be hypotonic.

H_2O +++

15 - The urine tends to be hypotonic

14 - Normally the excess water is distributed evenly throughout the ECF and the ICF. Plasma electrolytes and osmolarity are low

Untreated, the patient become confused, irritable, drowsy and then flaccidly comatose. **Water restriction** is the **treatment** although, in severe cases, an initial slow and small hypertonic infusion of 5% sodium chloride is indicated. If renal failure is present, this may demand dialysis.

18 - Untreated, the patient becomes confused, irritable and drowsy

17 - Treatment consists of water restriction but hypertonic infusion of 5% NaCl is indicated

16 - Flaccidity is also present

A low serum sodium (hyponatraemia) is also found where sodium depletion is the primary deficit – particularly in Addison's disease or the too vigorous use of diuretics. **Clinically** weakness or languor and apathy may be accompanied by cramps and sometimes vomiting and also hypovolaemic features of combined salt and water loss described above. **Specific treatment** of the underlying disorder is accompanied by saline replacement as both salt and water will be required. A patient with severe sodium deficiency may require 7-10 litres of physiological saline at first by rapid infusion and then more gradually, perhaps with CVP monitoring. Where the patient is very hyponatraemic, again a small and slow infusion of hypertonic saline may be used initially. Some advanced cardiac disease patients develop refractory hyponatraemia with peripheral oedema and are very difficult to treat.

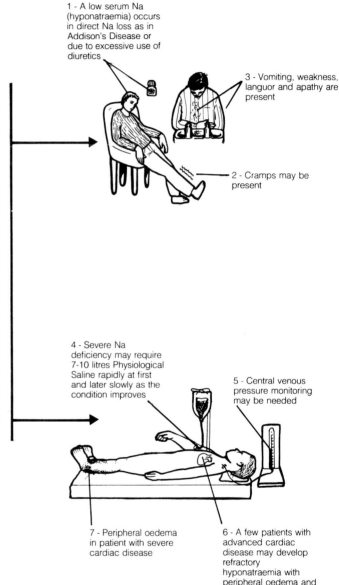

1 - A low serum Na (hyponatraemia) occurs in direct Na loss as in Addison's Disease or due to excessive use of diuretics

3 - Vomiting, weakness, languor and apathy are present

2 - Cramps may be present

4 - Severe Na deficiency may require 7-10 litres Physiological Saline rapidly at first and later slowly as the condition improves

5 - Central venous pressure monitoring may be needed

7 - Peripheral oedema in patient with severe cardiac disease

6 - A few patients with advanced cardiac disease may develop refractory hyponatraemia with peripheral oedema and are difficult to treat

Potassium: Potassium is the major intracellular cation and only 1-2% of the total body potassium is in the **ECF**. Thus plasma levels of potassium (normally 3.5–5.0 mMol/l) do not necessarily reflect whole body potassium status. An electrocardiogram (**ECG**) may often provide important information concerning intracellular potassium levels. In **hyperkalaemia**,(excessive blood potassium) the **ECG** demonstrates a tall and peaked T wave with a widened QRS complex and reduced R wave amplitude. In hypokalaemia, there is T wave flattening and an increasingly prominent U wave appears, (often mistaken for the T wave); the PR interval lengthens and there is depression of the ST segment. More sophisticated methods of measuring whole body potassium status exist but are not routinely available.

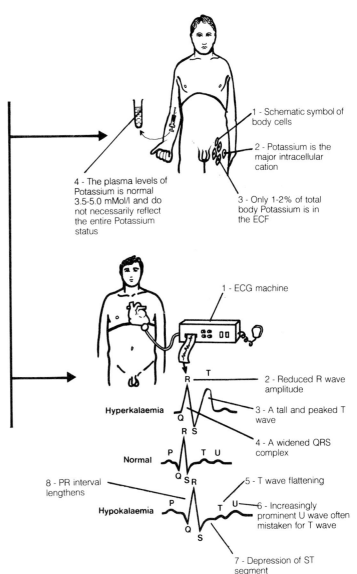

1 - Schematic symbol of body cells

2 - Potassium is the major intracellular cation

4 - The plasma levels of Potassium is normal 3.5-5.0 mMol/l and do not necessarily reflect the entire Potassium status

3 - Only 1-2% of total body Potassium is in the ECF

1 - ECG machine

2 - Reduced R wave amplitude

3 - A tall and peaked T wave

4 - A widened QRS complex

5 - T wave flattening

8 - PR interval lengthens

6 - Increasingly prominent U wave often mistaken for T wave

7 - Depression of ST segment

Hyperkalaemia

Normal

Hypokalaemia

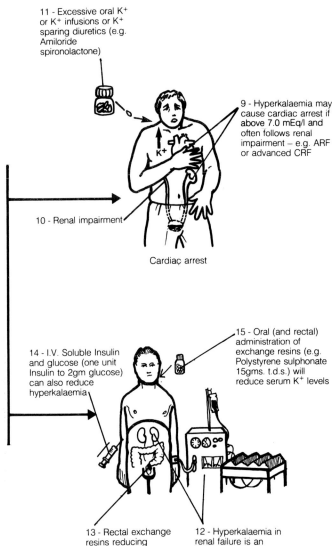

11 - Excessive oral K⁺ or K⁺ infusions or K⁺ sparing diuretics (e.g. Amiloride spironolactone)

9 - Hyperkalaemia may cause cardiac arrest if above 7.0 mEq/l and often follows renal impairment – e.g. ARF or advanced CRF

10 - Renal impairment

Cardiac arrest

14 - I.V. Soluble Insulin and glucose (one unit Insulin to 2gm glucose) can also reduce hyperkalaemia

15 - Oral (and rectal) administration of exchange resins (e.g. Polystyrene sulphonate 15gms. t.d.s.) will reduce serum K⁺ levels

13 - Rectal exchange resins reducing hyperkalaemia

12 - Hyperkalaemia in renal failure is an indication for dialysis

Hyperkalaemia may cause a cardiac arrest if above 7.0 mEq/l. Hyperkalaemia occurs most often following renal impairment (acute renal failure and advanced chronic renal failure) but also occurs iatrogenically by too rapid potassium infusions or excessive oral potassium supplements perhaps together with potassium sparing diuretics (e.g amiloride, spironolactone). Hyperkalaemia in renal failure is an indication for dialysis but a rapid reduction in the blood level can be effected by intravenous soluble insulin and glucose (in the proportion: one unit to two grams of glucose). Oral or rectal administration of an exchange resin (e.g. polystyrene sulphonate 15g tds), will also reduce serum levels.

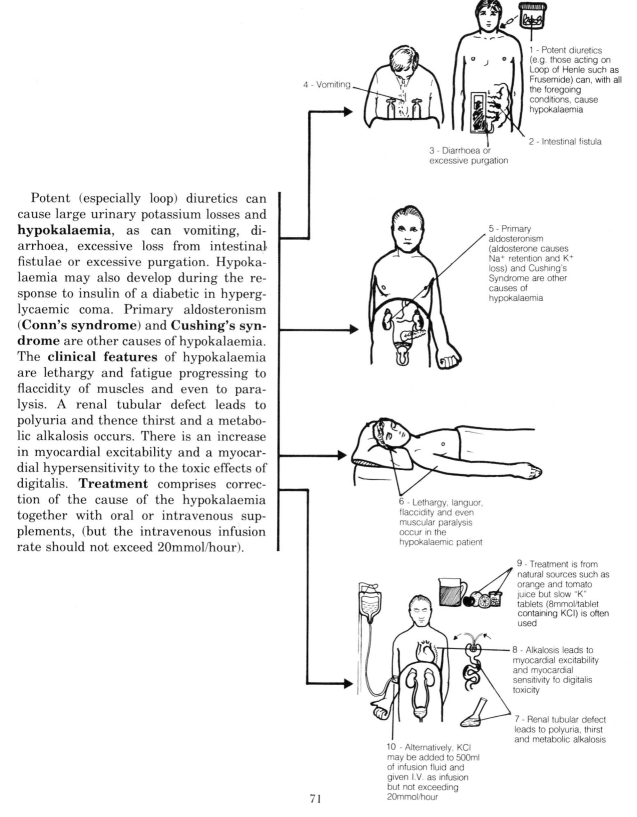

1 - Potent diuretics (e.g. those acting on Loop of Henle such as Frusemide) can, with all the foregoing conditions, cause hypokalaemia

2 - Intestinal fistula

3 - Diarrhoea or excessive purgation

4 - Vomiting

5 - Primary aldosteronism (aldosterone causes Na^+ retention and K^+ loss) and Cushing's Syndrome are other causes of hypokalaemia

6 - Lethargy, languor, flaccidity and even muscular paralysis occur in the hypokalaemic patient

9 - Treatment is from natural sources such as orange and tomato juice but slow "K" tablets (8mmol/tablet containing KCl) is often used

8 - Alkalosis leads to myocardial excitability and myocardial sensitivity fo digitalis toxicity

7 - Renal tubular defect leads to polyuria, thirst and metabolic alkalosis

10 - Alternatively, KCl may be added to 500ml of infusion fluid and given I.V. as infusion but not exceeding 20mmol/hour

Potent (especially loop) diuretics can cause large urinary potassium losses and **hypokalaemia**, as can vomiting, diarrhoea, excessive loss from intestinal fistulae or excessive purgation. Hypokalaemia may also develop during the response to insulin of a diabetic in hyperglycaemic coma. Primary aldosteronism (**Conn's syndrome**) and **Cushing's syndrome** are other causes of hypokalaemia. The **clinical features** of hypokalaemia are lethargy and fatigue progressing to flaccidity of muscles and even to paralysis. A renal tubular defect leads to polyuria and thence thirst and a metabolic alkalosis occurs. There is an increase in myocardial excitability and a myocardial hypersensitivity to the toxic effects of digitalis. **Treatment** comprises correction of the cause of the hypokalaemia together with oral or intravenous supplements, (but the intravenous infusion rate should not exceed 20mmol/hour).

Magnesium – Like Potassium, magnesium is mainly an intracellular cation whole plasma level is fixed normally at 0.7-1.2 mmol/litre, largely by unknown homeostatic mechanisms but related to calcium metabolism. Hypomagnesaemia may occur from heavy magnesium loss from gut or urine (e.g. malabsorption states, vomiting, excessive use of diuretics). **Clinical features** include muscle weakness, tetany, cardiac arrhythmias, vomiting and mental confusion. Oral magnesium hydroxide or intravenous magnesium chloride (not faster than 0.5mmol/min) is the treatment. Hypermagnesaemia is rare but may occur in CRF and contribute to the neuromuscular complications; magnesium containing preparations should be avoided in these patients.

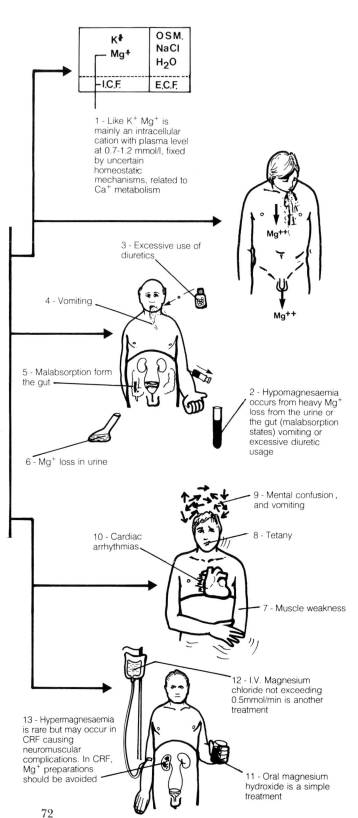

1 - Like K^+ Mg^+ is mainly an intracellular cation with plasma level at 0.7-1.2 mmol/l, fixed by uncertain homeostatic mechanisms, related to Ca^+ metabolism

3 - Excessive use of diuretics

4 - Vomiting

5 - Malabsorption form the gut

6 - Mg^+ loss in urine

2 - Hypomagnesaemia occurs from heavy Mg^+ loss from the urine or the gut (malabsorption states) vomiting or excessive diuretic usage

9 - Mental confusion, and vomiting

10 - Cardiac arrhythmias

8 - Tetany

7 - Muscle weakness

12 - I.V. Magnesium chloride not exceeding 0.5mmol/min is another treatment

13 - Hypermagnesaemia is rare but may occur in CRF causing neuromuscular complications. In CRF, Mg^+ preparations should be avoided

11 - Oral magnesium hydroxide is a simple treatment

ACID-BASE BALANCE

The **pH** of **ECF** is normally 7.4 (7.36-7.42) and this pH is tightly, homeostatically controlled, despite an innate and constant tendency towards metabolic acidosis caused by the perpetual production of hydrogen ions during metabolism. This tendency is minimised by the blood buffering systems which serve to reduce the "expected" pH change consequent upon adding H^+ (or OH^-) ions to the system. The final blood pH depends upon the ratio of buffer base to buffer acid thus:

$$pH = pK + \log \frac{(\text{Buffer base})}{(\text{Buffer acid})}$$
(Henderson Hasselbalch Equation)

The most important buffering system in the blood is the carbon dioxide – bicarbonate – carbonic acid system ($HCO_3^- + H^+ = H_2CO_3 = H_2O + CO_2$), for which $pH = 6.1 + \log \frac{(HCO_3^-)}{(H_2CO_3)}$. This buffering system can quickly compensate for pH changes as CO_2 can be rapidly excreted by the lungs.

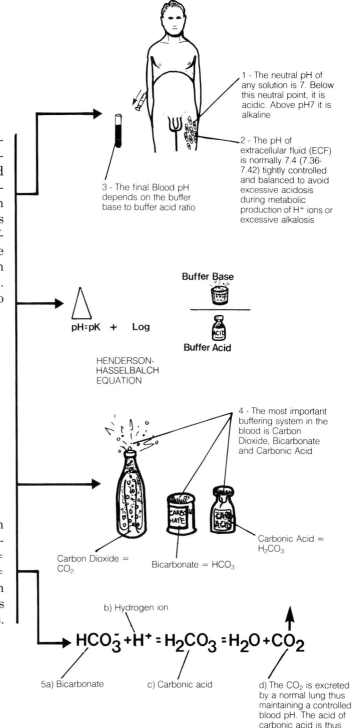

1 - The neutral pH of any solution is 7. Below this neutral point, it is acidic. Above pH7 it is alkaline

2 - The pH of extracellular fluid (ECF) is normally 7.4 (7.36-7.42) tightly controlled and balanced to avoid excessive acidosis during metabolic production of H^+ ions or excessive alkalosis

3 - The final Blood pH depends on the buffer base to buffer acid ratio

Buffer Base

Buffer Acid

$$pH = pK + Log$$

HENDERSON-HASSELBALCH EQUATION

4 - The most important buffering system in the blood is Carbon Dioxide, Bicarbonate and Carbonic Acid

Carbonic Acid = H_2CO_3

Carbon Dioxide = CO_2

Bicarbonate = HCO_3

b) Hydrogen ion

$$HCO_3^- + H^+ = H_2CO_3 = H_2O + CO_2$$

5a) Bicarbonate

c) Carbonic acid

d) The CO_2 is excreted by a normal lung thus maintaining a controlled blood pH. The acid of carbonic acid is thus removed from the blood

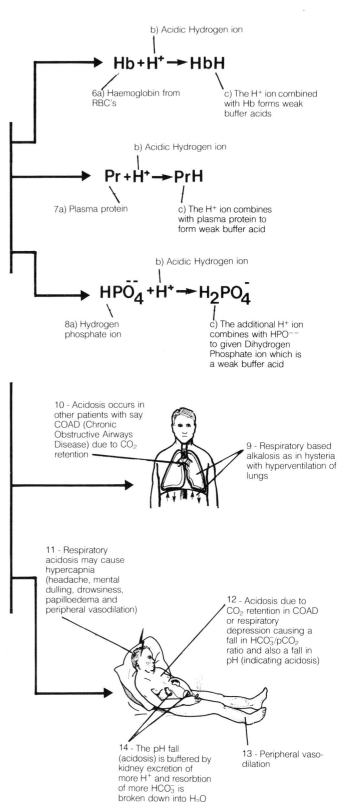

b) Acidic Hydrogen ion

$$Hb + H^+ \rightarrow HbH$$

6a) Haemoglobin from RBC's

c) The H$^+$ ion combined with Hb forms weak buffer acids

b) Acidic Hydrogen ion

$$Pr + H^+ \rightarrow PrH$$

7a) Plasma protein

c) The H$^+$ ion combines with plasma protein to form weak buffer acid

b) Acidic Hydrogen ion

$$HPO_4^{--} + H^+ \rightarrow H_2PO_4^-$$

8a) Hydrogen phosphate ion

c) The additional H$^+$ ion combines with HPO^{--} to given Dihydrogen Phosphate ion which is a weak buffer acid

Other "interconnected" blood buffering systems include haemoglobin, plasma proteins and phosphate. If the respiratory function is normal then the plasma bicarbonate concentration indicates the total available buffer base. However, in respiratory based alkalosis or acidosis, this is not so and arterial pH and pCO_2 (normal range 36-42mmHg) are necessary investigations to quantify the defect.

Respiratory acidosis is most commonly due to alveolar hypoventilation (as in advanced **COAD** or direct respiratory depression) leading to CO_2 retention, a fall in the $\frac{HCO_2}{pCO_2}$ ratio and consequently a fall in pH. The pH fall is buffered to some degree by the other blood buffering systems and the kidney excretes more H$^+$ and reabsorbs more HCO$^-_3$ in an attempt to compensate. The clinical picture of respiratory acidosis is usually a complex one with features of both hypercapnia (headache, mental dulling, drowsiness, papilloedema, peripheral vasodilation) and hypoxia.

10 - Acidosis occurs in other patients with say COAD (Chronic Obstructive Airways Disease) due to CO_2 retention

9 - Respiratory based alkalosis as in hysteria with hyperventilation of lungs

11 - Respiratory acidosis may cause hypercapnia (headache, mental dulling, drowsiness, papilloedema and peripheral vasodilation)

12 - Acidosis due to CO_2 retention in COAD or respiratory depression causing a fall in HCO$^-_3$/pCO$_2$ ratio and also a fall in pH (indicating acidosis)

14 - The pH fall (acidosis) is buffered by kidney excretion of more H$^+$ and resorbtion of more HCO$^-_3$ is broken down into H$_2$O and CO$_2$

13 - Peripheral vasodilation

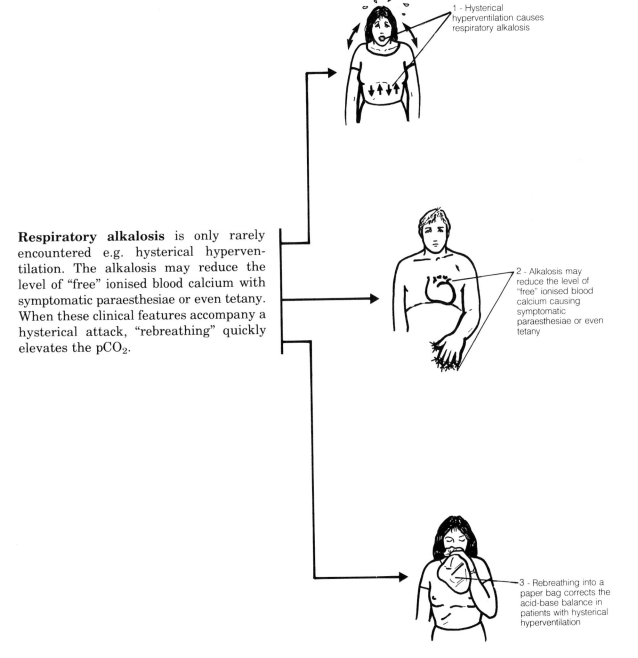

1 - Hysterical hyperventilation causes respiratory alkalosis

2 - Alkalosis may reduce the level of "free" ionised blood calcium causing symptomatic paraesthesiae or even tetany

3 - Rebreathing into a paper bag corrects the acid-base balance in patients with hysterical hyperventilation

Respiratory alkalosis is only rarely encountered e.g. hysterical hyperventilation. The alkalosis may reduce the level of "free" ionised blood calcium with symptomatic paraesthesiae or even tetany. When these clinical features accompany a hysterical attack, "rebreathing" quickly elevates the pCO$_2$.

Metabolic acidosis is usually due to the additon of some acid to the system – e.g.. keto – acids in diabetic coma, the ingestion of acid or acid producing substances such as aspirin or ammonium chloride, enhanced production of lactic acid during tissue hypoxia (e.g after severe exercise or after cardiac arrest), or due to the failure to excrete acid products of metabolism as in CRF, (and renal tubular acidosis). The **clinical sign** of metabolic acidosis is hyperventilation, (a compensating pulmonary mechanism exploiting the $HCO_3-H_2CO_3-CO_2$ system to its full capacity). Other clinical features are weakness and tiredness. **Treatment** is of the underlying condition and reversing any factors embarrassing renal function.

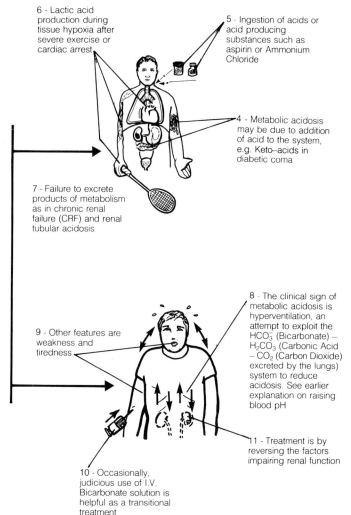

6 - Lactic acid production during tissue hypoxia after severe exercise or cardiac arrest

5 - Ingestion of acids or acid producing substances such as aspirin or Ammonium Chloride

4 - Metabolic acidosis may be due to addition of acid to the system, e.g. Keto–acids in diabetic coma

7 - Failure to excrete products of metabolism as in chronic renal failure (CRF) and renal tubular acidosis

8 - The clinical sign of metabolic acidosis is hyperventilation, an attempt to exploit the HCO_3^- (Bicarbonate) – H_2CO_3 (Carbonic Acid) – CO_2 (Carbon Dioxide) excreted by the lungs) system to reduce acidosis. See earlier explanation on raising blood pH

9 - Other features are weakness and tiredness

11 - Treatment is by reversing the factors impairing renal function

10 - Occasionally, judicious use of I.V. Bicarbonate solution is helpful as a transitional treatment

Occasionally judicious use of intravenous bicarbonate solution is indicated as an interim measure.

Metabolic alkalosis is encountered following prolonged vomiting of (acidic) gastric contents, when there is always concomitant salt and water depletion. Compensatory hypoventilation is rarely evident and treatment is of the underlying disorder with correction of saline depletion, whereupon renal regulation soon returns the system to normal. Renal potassium losses may increase during this renal conservation of hydrogen ions, and hypokalaemia should be watched for and corrected; (conversely, hypokalaemia may lead to a metabolic alkalosis!).

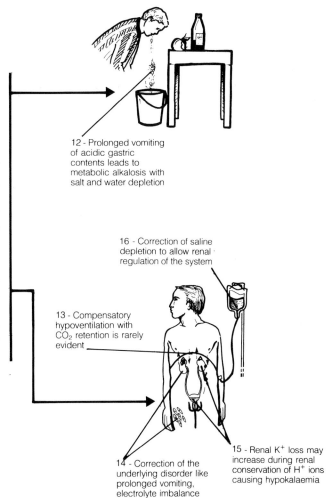

12 - Prolonged vomiting of acidic gastric contents leads to metabolic alkalosis with salt and water depletion

16 - Correction of saline depletion to allow renal regulation of the system

13 - Compensatory hypoventilation with CO_2 retention is rarely evident

14 - Correction of the underlying disorder like prolonged vomiting, electrolyte imbalance and dehydration

15 - Renal K^+ loss may increase during renal conservation of H^+ ions causing hypokalaemia

Poisoning

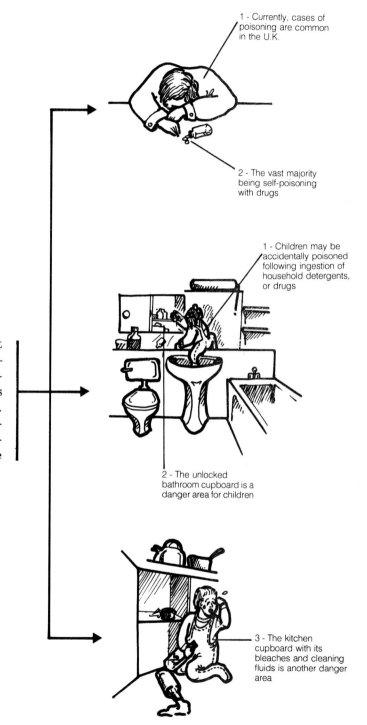

1 - Currently, cases of poisoning are common in the U.K.

2 - The vast majority being self-poisoning with drugs

1 - Children may be accidentally poisoned following ingestion of household detergents, or drugs

2 - The unlocked bathroom cupboard is a danger area for children

3 - The kitchen cupboard with its bleaches and cleaning fluids is another danger area

DRUG POISONING

In clinical medicine in the U.K. at present cases of poisoning are common — the vast majority of cases being self-poisoning with drugs, either as serious suicide attempts or as a "cry of help". Children may become accidentally poisoned following ingestion of household products, (bleach, disinfectant, anti-freeze

1 - Less common are poisonings due to industrial chemicals or radio-isotopes and from heavy metals

etc.), or drugs. Less common are poisonings due to industrial chemicals or radio-isotopes and from heavy metals. Homicidal poisonings are rare but must be borne in mind where a diagnosis is lacking. Snake venom, insect stings, berries and other vegetable matter provide a "natural" form of poisoning.

2 - Snake venom, insect stings, berries and other vegetable matter provide 'natural' poisons

In many severe drug poisonings there may be depressed consciousness and, with the deeper levels of coma, depressed spontaneous respiration. Additionally, there may be hypotension and hypovolaemic shock with pre-renal failure. For this reason, the first step in the management of a patient admitted with drug poisoning is to assess the level of consciousness, (see illustrated lecture series: Neurology Section: 'COMA'), the respiratory drive (with arterial gas measurements) and the cardiovascular status, (pulse, blood pressure, peripheral perfusion). In comatose patients an airway is ensured by suction of the pharynx and by nursing the patient in the tonsillar position with an oropharyngeal airway *in situ*. If spontaneous respiration is inadequate, then mechanical ventilation will be necessary and a cuffed endotracheal tube is inserted. If there is cardiovascular collapse, then a head down position is adopted until a CVP line is in place and a colloid infusion together with an inotropic drug (isoprenaline, dubotamine) is under way. Even if the coma, respiration and cardiovascular systems are not critically embarrassed on admission, these systems must be frequently monitored until the danger is past.

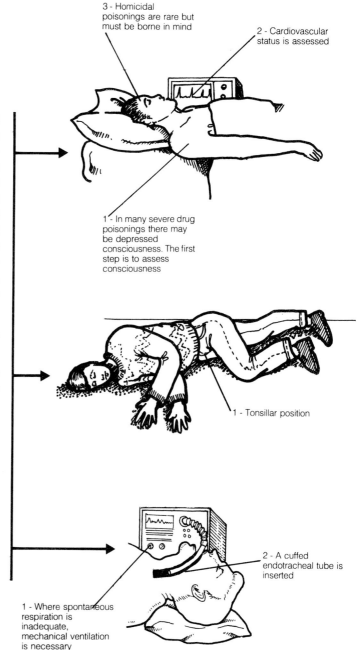

3 - Homicidal poisonings are rare but must be borne in mind

2 - Cardiovascular status is assessed

1 - In many severe drug poisonings there may be depressed consciousness. The first step is to assess consciousness

1 - Tonsillar position

1 - Where spontaneous respiration is inadequate, mechanical ventilation is necessary

2 - A cuffed endotracheal tube is inserted

Having established this first priority supportive therapy, the clinician next requires to know from the patient, witnesses or other clues (e.g. empty drug containers), what drug has been ingested by what route, in what quantity and how long ago? Blood is drawn for serum levels of suspected drugs and for "umbrella analysis" if the drug is unknown. For drugs ingested orally within four hours of admission, the stomach should be emptied of its contents. For salicylate poisoning and poisoning by drugs likely to delay gastric emptying (e.g tricyclic antidepressants, anticholinergics), the stomach may be productively emptied up to 16 hours after the poisoning.

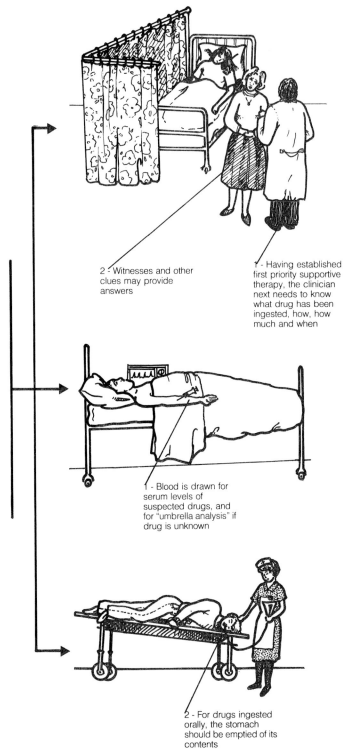

2 - Witnesses and other clues may provide answers

1 - Having established first priority supportive therapy, the clinician next needs to know what drug has been ingested, how, how much and when

1 - Blood is drawn for serum levels of suspected drugs, and for "umbrella analysis" if drug is unknown

2 - For drugs ingested orally, the stomach should be emptied of its contents

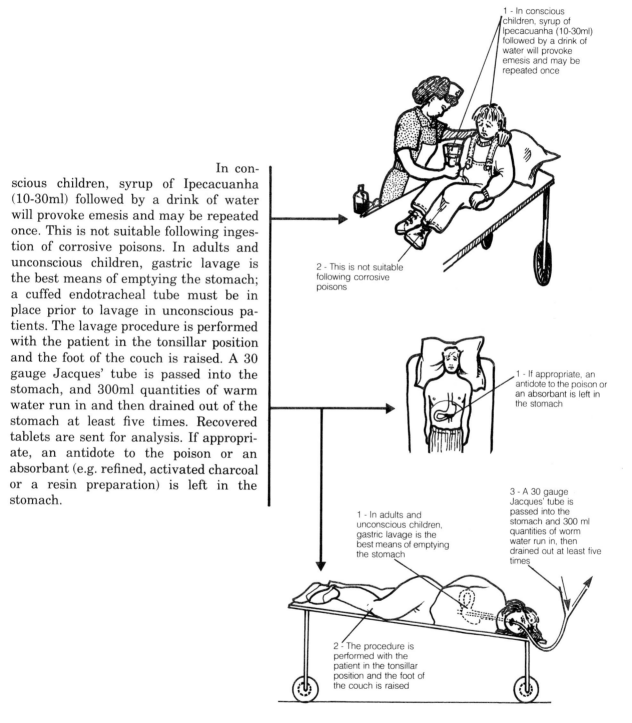

1 - In conscious children, syrup of Ipecacuanha (10-30ml) followed by a drink of water will provoke emesis and may be repeated once

2 - This is not suitable following corrosive poisons

1 - If appropriate, an antidote to the poison or an absorbant is left in the stomach

3 - A 30 gauge Jacques' tube is passed into the stomach and 300 ml quantities of worm water run in, then drained out at least five times

1 - In adults and unconscious children, gastric lavage is the best means of emptying the stomach

2 - The procedure is performed with the patient in the tonsillar position and the foot of the couch is raised

In conscious children, syrup of Ipecacuanha (10-30ml) followed by a drink of water will provoke emesis and may be repeated once. This is not suitable following ingestion of corrosive poisons. In adults and unconscious children, gastric lavage is the best means of emptying the stomach; a cuffed endotracheal tube must be in place prior to lavage in unconscious patients. The lavage procedure is performed with the patient in the tonsillar position and the foot of the couch is raised. A 30 gauge Jacques' tube is passed into the stomach, and 300ml quantities of warm water run in and then drained out of the stomach at least five times. Recovered tablets are sent for analysis. If appropriate, an antidote to the poison or an absorbant (e.g. refined, activated charcoal or a resin preparation) is left in the stomach.

Specific **antidotes** are available against certain drugs. In opiate poisoning (morphine, heroin/diamorphine, pethidine, methadone), naloxone (0.4mg i.v. state, repeated in five minutes and again as required), is a specific antidote. Methionine or N-acetyl cysteine are antidotes in paracetamol poisoning, Berlin blue inactivates thallium, cobalt edetate inactivates cyanides and oxygen counteracts carbon monoxide gas poisoning. Antivenom is available for some snake bites.

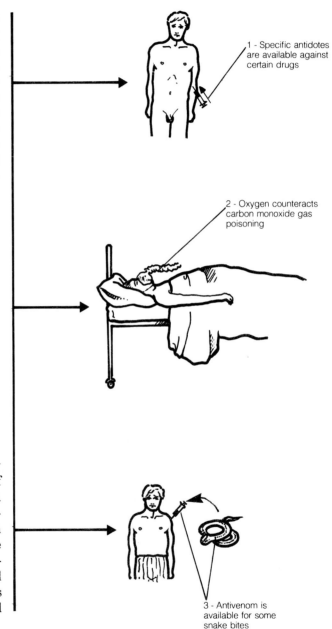

1 - Specific antidotes are available against certain drugs

2 - Oxygen counteracts carbon monoxide gas poisoning

3 - Antivenom is available for some snake bites

In some types of drug poisoning it may be possible to enhance the elimination of the poison. **Forced alkaline diuresis** is a technique useful for drugs largely excreted unchanged by the kidneys and which tend to dissociate into their ionised state more readily in alkaline pH, (thus reducing their reabsorption from the renal tubules). Such drugs include salicylates and phenobarbitone. In patients poisoned by these agents and who have normal renal function, a urine flow of 500ml/hour is produced by intravenous infusions of standard crystalloid preparations (0.9% saline and dextrose saline) and the pH of the urine is raised to 7.5 – 8.5 by sodium bicarbonate infusion. Plasma electrolytes (especially potassium) must be carefully monitored during alkaline diuresis.

1 - Intravenous infusions of standard crystalloid preparations

For other drugs, methods of enhanced elimination are less easy but dialysable drugs can be removed by haemodialysis. This is usually impracticable but haemoperfusion is possible in some poisons' units. This technique involves the setting up of an extracorporeal blood circuit, the blood flowing through a column of sterile adsorbent, (activated charcoal or non-ionic resin), before returning to the body. The results of haemoperfusion have been impressive in some cases of barbiturate poisoning.

1 - Dialysis drugs can be removed by haemodialysis but this is impracticable

2 - Haemoperfusion is possible in some poisons' units

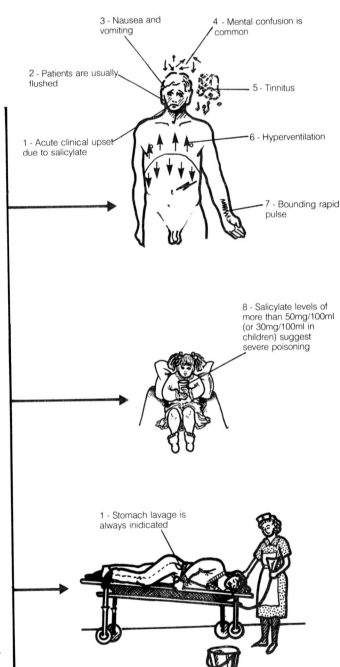

Particular Acute Drug Poisoning Problems

a) **Salicylates** – The acute clinical upset involves nausea and vomiting, tinnitus and hyperventilation (compensatory for the metabolic acidosis). Patients are usually flushed due to vasodilatation with a bounding rapid pulse. Mental confusion is common. Severe poisoning may be suspected if admission or subsequent blood samples give plasma salicylate levels of more than 50mg/100ml, (or 30mg/100ml in children).

The principles of therapy have been documented above; stomach lavage is always indicated and for poisonings more than a "token overdose" forced alkaline diuresis is commenced. In very serious poisonings with renal and circulatory failure, haemoperfusion is indicated. Vitamin K, injections may reduce the bleeding tendency.

b) **Paracetamol** – Paracetamol depends on hepatic degradation for its elimination. A small proportion of hepatic catabolite comprises a potent hepatotoxin. In the presence of the naturally occurring hepatic glutathione, this hepatotoxin will be neutralised but in a severe acute drug overdosage (more than 15-20g), the glutathione is overwhelmed and fatal liver damage may occur.

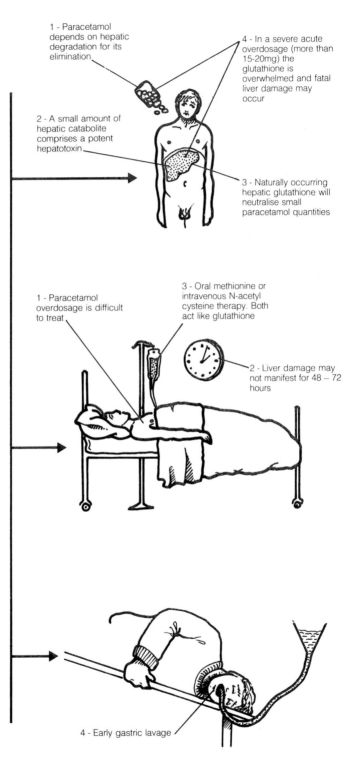

1 - Paracetamol depends on hepatic degradation for its elimination

2 - A small amount of hepatic catabolite comprises a potent hepatotoxin

3 - Naturally occurring hepatic glutathione will neutralise small paracetamol quantities

4 - In a severe acute overdosage (more than 15-20mg) the glutathione is overwhelmed and fatal liver damage may occur

1 - Paracetamol overdosage is difficult to treat

3 - Oral methionine or intravenous N-acetyl cysteine therapy. Both act like glutathione

2 - Liver damage may not manifest for 48 – 72 hours

4 - Early gastric lavage

Paracetamol overdosage is difficult to treat and liver damage may not manifest for 48–72 hours. Early gastric lavage and oral methionine or intravenous N-acetyl cysteine therapy, (both of which act like glutathione, due to their sulphydryl groups), are the mainstays of therapy. A

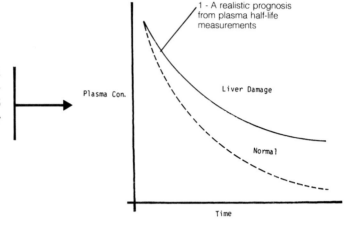

1 - A realistic prognosis from plasma half-life measurements

Plasma Con.

Liver Damage

Normal

Time

realistic prognosis may be obtained from plasma paracetamol half-life measurements – a plasma half-life in excess of 4-6 hours represents potentially fatal liver poisoning.

c) **Tricyclic Antidepressants** – The clinical picture of acute overdosage may commence with excitability prior to CNS depression, coma, even convulsions. Cardiovascular effects are important in tricyclic overdosage, hypotension may be early and tachydysrhythmias may be life threatening. All patients require cardiac monitoring and appropriate anti-dysrhythmic therapy plus circulatory support with plasma expanders. Physostigmine (1-3mg) i.v. slow bolus may counteract CNS and cardiovascular effects.

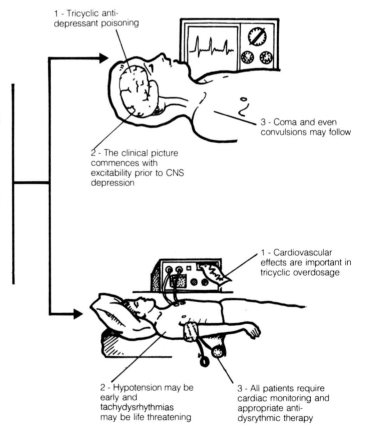

1 - Tricyclic anti-depressant poisoning

2 - The clinical picture commences with excitability prior to CNS depression

3 - Coma and even convulsions may follow

1 - Cardiovascular effects are important in tricyclic overdosage

2 - Hypotension may be early and tachydysrhythmias may be life threatening

3 - All patients require cardiac monitoring and appropriate anti-dysrythmic therapy

Regrettably, neither forced diuresis nor dialysis are effective at enhancing elimination and treatment is entirely supportive.

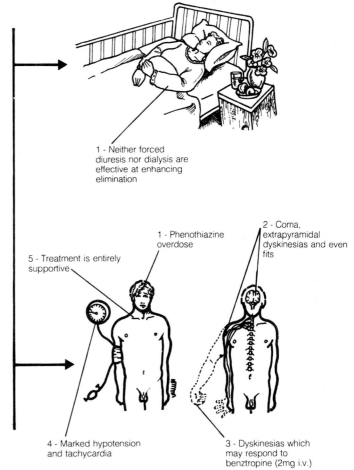

1 - Neither forced diuresis nor dialysis are effective at enhancing elimination

5 - Treatment is entirely supportive

1 - Phenothiazine overdose

2 - Coma, extrapyramidal dyskinesias and even fits

4 - Marked hypotension and tachycardia

3 - Dyskinesias which may respond to benztropine (2mg i.v.)

d) **Phenothiazines** – Phenothiazine overdosage produces coma, extrapyramidal dyskinesias and even fits, and marked hypotension and tachycardia, (due to adrenergic blocking actions). Treatment is supportive; dyskinesias may respond to benztropine (2mg i.v.).

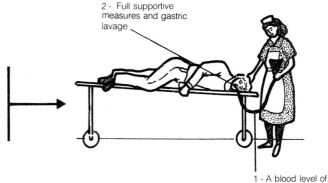

2 - Full supportive measures and gastric lavage

1 - A blood level of 300mg per 100ml is dangerous to life and levels approaching this require intervention

e) **Ethyl Alcohol** – A blood level of 300mg per 100ml is dangerous to life and levels approaching this require active intervention with full supportive measures and gastric lavage. An intravenous

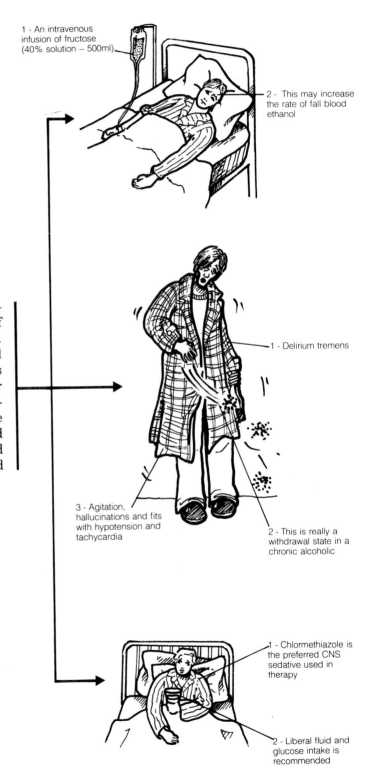

1 - An intravenous infusion of fructose (40% solution – 500ml)

2 - This may increase the rate of fall blood ethanol

1 - Delirium tremens

2 - This is really a withdrawal state in a chronic alcoholic

3 - Agitation, hallucinations and fits with hypotension and tachycardia

1 - Chlormethiazole is the preferred CNS sedative used in therapy

2 - Liberal fluid and glucose intake is recommended

infusion of fructose (40% solution – 500ml), may increase the rate of fall of blood ethanol. Dialysis may be necessary. **Delirium tremens** is really a withdrawal state in a chronic alcoholic and comprises agitation, hallucinations and fits together with hypotension and tachycardia. Chlormethiazole is the preferred CNS sedative used in therapy and a liberal fluid and glucose intake is recommended. Blood electrolyte (including magnesium) and glucose levels should be monitored. A Vitamin B, (thiamine rich) and C formulation is commenced intravenously.

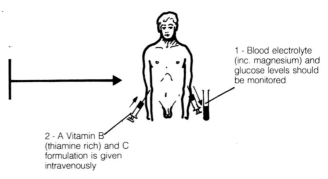

1 - Blood electrolyte (inc. magnesium) and glucose levels should be monitored

2 - A Vitamin B (thiamine rich) and C formulation is given intravenously

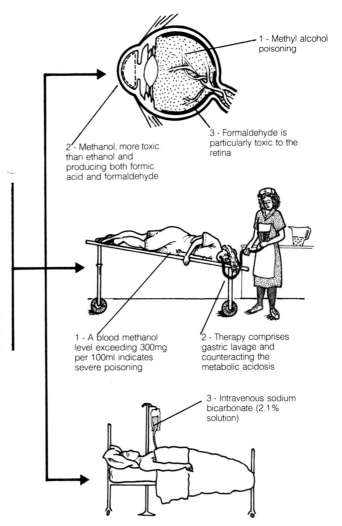

1 - Methyl alcohol poisoning

2 - Methanol, more toxic than ethanol and producing both formic acid and formaldehyde

3 - Formaldehyde is particularly toxic to the retina

f) **Methyl Alcohol** – Methanol is more toxic than ethanol and both formic acid and formaldehyde are produced in its metabolism. Formaldehyde is particularly toxic to the retina. A blood methanol level exceeding 300mg per 100ml indicates severe poisoning. Therapy comprises gastric lavage and counteracting the metabolic acidosis with intravenous sodium bicarbonate (2.1% solution). Blood electrolytes must be monitored. The

1 - A blood methanol level exceeding 300mg per 100ml indicates severe poisoning

2 - Therapy comprises gastric lavage and counteracting the metabolic acidosis

3 - Intravenous sodium bicarbonate (2.1% solution)

metabolism of methanol, (and hence the accumulation of toxic catabolites), may be slowed by the administration of ethanol, (50%, 1ml/kg orally stat and 0.5ml/kg two hourly for five days). If vision is already impaired, or renal failure occurs, dialysis is indicated.

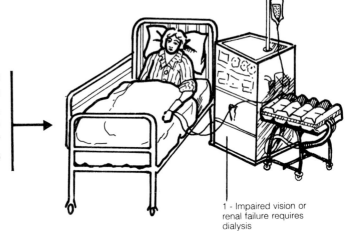

1 - Impaired vision or renal failure requires dialysis

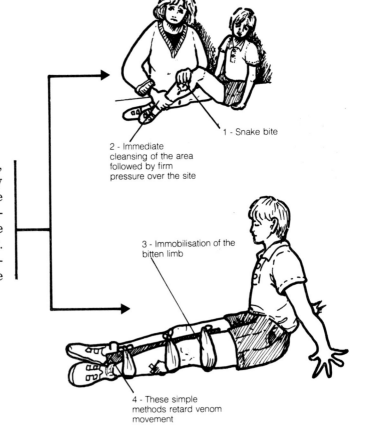

1 - Snake bite

2 - Immediate cleansing of the area followed by firm pressure over the site

3 - Immobilisation of the bitten limb

4 - These simple methods retard venom movement

g) **Snake Bites** – Following a snake bite, cleansing the area should be followed by firm pressure over the site of the bite together with immobilisation of the bitten limb, usually by splinting. These simple methods retard venom movement. Arterial tourniquets are no longer recommended. Anti-venoms are available against some snake bites but, where appropriate, effective therapy must involve the early systemic administration of liberal quantities of the anti-venom.

(**N.B.** Anti-venoms are foreign proteins and anaphylaxis may occur following their administration. A small test injection should precede the full dose).

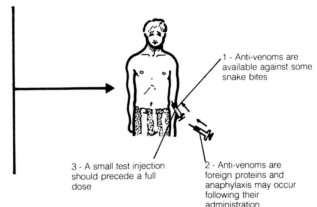

1 - Anti-venoms are available against some snake bites

3 - A small test injection should precede a full dose

2 - Anti-venoms are foreign proteins and anaphylaxis may occur following their administration

FOOD POISONING

"Food poisoning" is a lay term but useful to describe a number of illnesses where gastrointestinal symptoms arise within a day or so of eating a particular food – contaminated by bacteria, bacterial toxins or by chemicals. The term is confusing in that it does not embrace certain specific infections carried in food or water notably: typhoid fever, paratyphoid fever, bacillary dysentery, cholera, viral gastroenteritis, campylobacter enteritis, food allergy (e.g. to shellfish) etc. However, the term survives and the important causes are listed:–

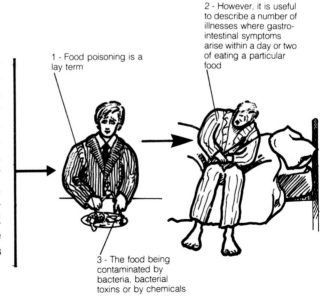

2 - However, it is useful to describe a number of illnesses where gastrointestinal symptoms arise within a day or two of eating a particular food

1 - Food poisoning is a lay term

3 - The food being contaminated by bacteria, bacterial toxins or by chemicals

Staphylococcal Food Poisoning –
Staph. aureus may produce an enterotoxin
and infected persons may contaminate
foodstuffs where the bacterium multiplies. Processed meats are common "culture
media". Within 1 – 6 hours of ingestion,
the patient experiences the sudden onset
of severe intestinal colic, vomiting and
diarrhoea. The attack is severe but for-
tunately usually short lasting and spontaneously remitting. Diagnosis comes
from the recovery of the bacterium in the
vomitus.

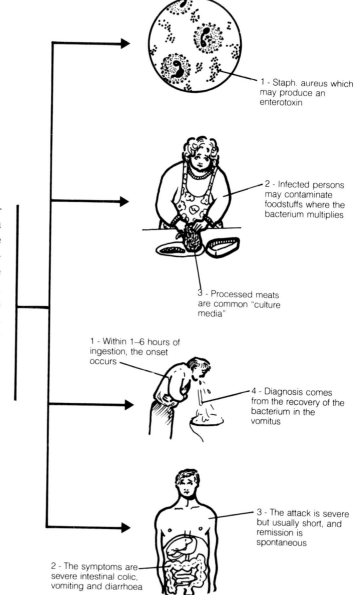

1 - Staph. aureus which
may produce an
enterotoxin

2 - Infected persons
may contaminate
foodstuffs where the
bacterium multiplies

3 - Processed meats
are common "culture
media"

1 - Within 1–6 hours of
ingestion, the onset
occurs

4 - Diagnosis comes
from the recovery of the
bacterium in the
vomitus

3 - The attack is severe
but usually short, and
remission is
spontaneous

2 - The symptoms are
severe intestinal colic,
vomiting and diarrhoea

1 - The treatment is symptomatic

3 - Antibiotics are usually unnecessary

2 - Adequate fluid replacement and anti-diarrhoeal agents

Treatment is symptomatic with adequate fluid replacement and antidiarrhoeal agents – antibiotics are usually unnecessary.

1 - Salmonella food poisoning

2 - S. typhimurium produces an acute gastro-enteritis

Salmonella Food Poisoning – In particular, *S. typhimurium* produces an acute gastroenteritis which occurs within two days of ingesting infected food. Vomiting, colic, diarrhoea are usually severe and a systemic upset with fever, malaise and even rigors may occur. Stool culture

4 - Vomiting, colic, diarrhoea are usually severe

3 - It occurs within 2 days of ingesting infected food

5 - Systemic upset with fever, malaise and even rigors may occur

provides the diagnosis and treatment comprises adquate fluid replacement and symptomatic therapy with anti-diarrhoeals. Antibiotics are probably unnecessary as the condition is usually self-terminating.

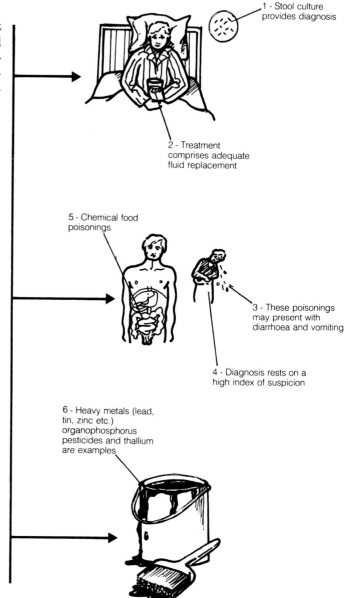

1 - Stool culture provides diagnosis

2 - Treatment comprises adequate fluid replacement

5 - Chemical food poisonings

3 - These poisonings may present with diarrhoea and vomiting

4 - Diagnosis rests on a high index of suspicion

6 - Heavy metals (lead, tin, zinc etc.) organophosphorus pesticides and thallium are examples

Chemical Food Poisoning – Heavy metals, (lead, tin, zinc etc.), organophosphorus pesticides and thallium are all examples of poisons that may present with diarrhoea and vomiting. Diagnosis rests on a high index of suspicion.

HAZARDS OF RADIATION AND RADIATION PROTECTION

Electromagnetic radiation is a form of energy propagated by wave motion; it ranges from radiowaves of long wavelength (3×10^4m) and low frequency (10^4 Hertz) to X-rays of short wavelength 10^{-12}m and high frequency (3×10^{20} Hertz). The high frequency X-rays are capable of causing ionising events in biological tissues (**ionising radiation**) and when these occur in DNA they may kill cells or create mutagenic events leading to late cancers or germ cell damage with genetic abnormalities. When "wave motion" radiation imparts this damage to biological tissue, it is better thought of as **Photon** radiation (which Einstein theory considers to be radiation comprised of packets of energy). Photon radiation derives from natural electromagnetic radiation sources in the solar system, from man-made X-ray sources, (for both diagnostic radiology and for therapy of cancer-radiotherapy), and from the ४ (gamma) emissions of naturally occurring radio-isotopes. The radiobiology of the interaction of X-rays and ४ rays with biological tissues is identical.

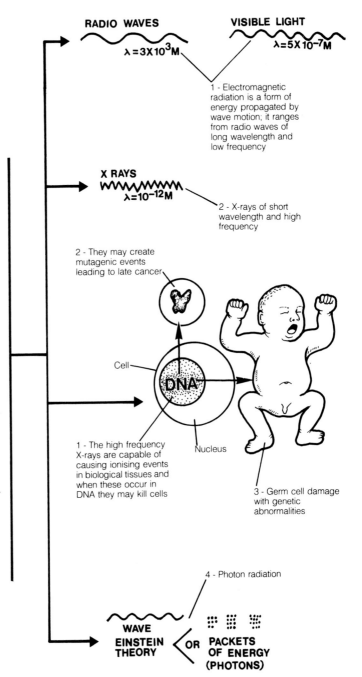

RADIO WAVES

$\lambda = 3 \times 10^3$M

VISIBLE LIGHT

$\lambda = 5 \times 10^{-7}$M

1 - Electromagnetic radiation is a form of energy propagated by wave motion; it ranges from radio waves of long wavelength and low frequency

X RAYS

$\lambda = 10^{-12}$M

2 - X-rays of short wavelength and high frequency

2 - They may create mutagenic events leading to late cancer

Cell

DNA

1 - The high frequency X-rays are capable of causing ionising events in biological tissues and when these occur in DNA they may kill cells

Nucleus

3 - Germ cell damage with genetic abnormalities

4 - Photon radiation

WAVE
EINSTEIN
THEORY

OR

PACKETS
OF ENERGY
(PHOTONS)

The decay of a radioactive isotope takes place exponentially as a function of time, to a more stable form; (the time to decay to one half-life of any initial value is known as the half-life: T½). The activity of a radioactive source is measured in disintegrations per second (units: The Curie, The Becquerel). When a radio isotope decays, not only may ४ (gamma) photons be emitted by ionising particulate radiation particles may be emitted (electrons or (Beta) ß particles, protons or ∝ (alpha) particles, neutrons, others). These radiation particles may have a greater biological effect than their radiation absorbed dose suggests – leading to the requirement of a quality factors (Q.F.) in radiation protection work.

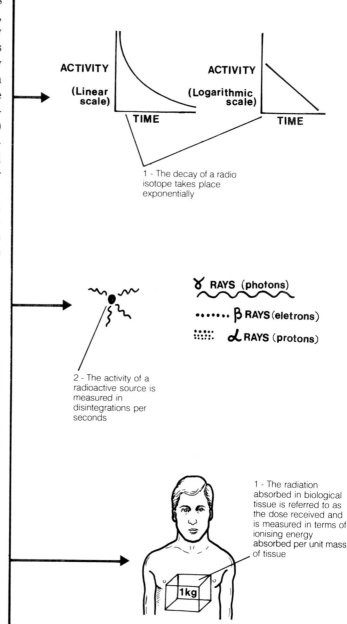

1 - The decay of a radio isotope takes place exponentially

2 - The activity of a radioactive source is measured in disintegrations per seconds

1 - The radiation absorbed in biological tissue is referred to as the dose received and is measured in terms of ionising energy absorbed per unit mass of tissue

The radiation absorbed in biological tissue is referred to as the dose received and is measured in terms of ionising energy absorbed per unit mass of tissue (units – one Gray equals one joule per kilogram) but because of the "greater than expected" biological effects of some radiation particle beams the unit used in radiation protection work is the Sievert which is related to the Gray by the following equation:–

Absorbed Radiation
"Equivalent" = Absorbed Dose
(Sievert) (Gray)
× Quality Factor
(e.g. × 1 for X-rays
× 10 for neutrons)

Following the disastrous radiation leaks from Three Mile Island (USA) and Chernobyl (USSR) nuclear power plants, the worldwide plutonium contamination following nuclear bombs, the increased use of radiation in medicine and other aspects of life, and contamination from natural radiation sources, it is essential that we have some idea of the risks, some ability to quantify those risks, and "dose limits".

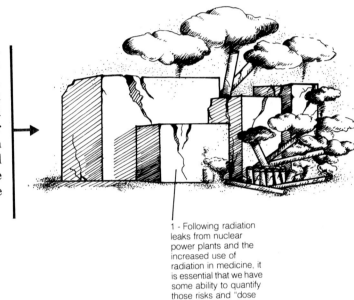

1 - Following radiation leaks from nuclear power plants and the increased use of radiation in medicine, it is essential that we have some ability to quantify those risks and "dose limits"

Maximum Permissible Dose

Since the effects of ionising radiation are cumulative, safe working conditions demand that the dose received should be as low as possible. It is unreasonable to say that the level of radiation should be zero as mankind has evolved in the presence of background cosmic radiaton and there is background terrestrial radiation all around us; it is also a fact of life now that man-made plutonium radio isotopes can be found in every corner of the world. The International Commission for

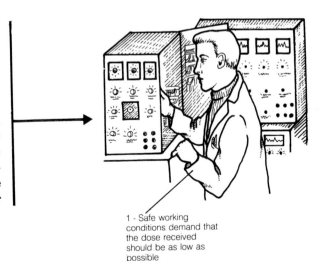

1 - Safe working conditions demand that the dose received should be as low as possible

Radiological Protection (ICRP) publish recommendations on what are "acceptable" upper limits of radiation that humans can receive and they express these maximum permissible doses in Sievert (old units – the rem). Workers in occupations which will be expected to be involved in work with radiation sources (eg. medical radiologists, nuclear power workers) are called: Designated workers. Designated workers are allowed to receive higher doses each year than the rest of the population but the doses received must be carefully monitored. In hospital service the "film badge" is the simplest monitoring device but a small portable ionising chamber dosimeter is more accurate.

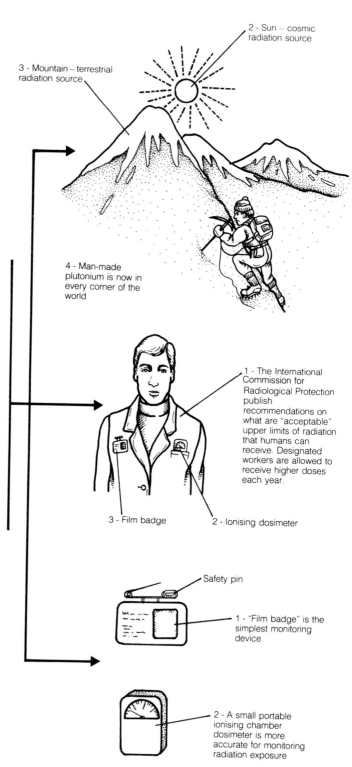

2 - Sun – cosmic radiation source

3 - Mountain – terrestrial radiation source

4 - Man-made plutonium is now in every corner of the world

1 - The International Commission for Radiological Protection publish recommendations on what are "acceptable" upper limits of radiation that humans can receive. Designated workers are allowed to receive higher doses each year.

3 - Film badge

2 - Ionising dosimeter

Safety pin

1 - "Film badge" is the simplest monitoring device

2 - A small portable ionising chamber dosimeter is more accurate for monitoring radiation exposure

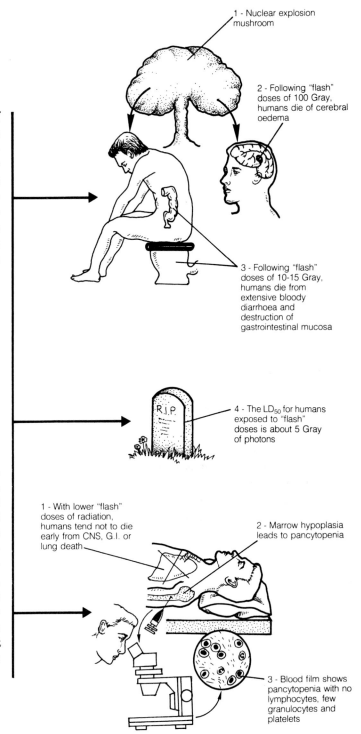

1 - Nuclear explosion mushroom

2 - Following "flash" doses of 100 Gray, humans die of cerebral oedema

3 - Following "flash" doses of 10-15 Gray, humans die from extensive bloody diarrhoea and destruction of gastrointestinal mucosa

4 - The LD_{50} for humans exposed to "flash" doses is about 5 Gray of photons

1 - With lower "flash" doses of radiation, humans tend not to die early from CNS, G.I. or lung death

2 - Marrow hypoplasia leads to pancytopenia

3 - Blood film shows pancytopenia with no lymphocytes, few granulocytes and platelets

Effects of Radiation Overdose

Following a "flash dose" of radiation of 100Gy, a human will die within six to twelve hours of cerebral swelling (oedema). Following "flash" doses of the order of 10-15 Gray, the human will die within the first week from extensive bloody diarrhoea and destruction of the gastrointestinal mucosa, or, should he survive this, from radiation pneumonitis, (which has a slightly longer latency of onset than G.I. death).

With lower "flash" doses of radiation, humans tend not to die early from CNS, G.I. or lung death, but to die from bone marrow hypoplasia or aplasia with a mean time to death of 30 days. From the Hiroshima and Nagasaki data, the estimated median lethal dose (LD_{50}) for marrow death in humans is said to 4.5 Gray, but with modern hospital methods of bone marrow support, (and the failure of Quality Factors to be taken into full account in the Japanese data), this probably means that the human LD_{50} to "flash" dose radiation is approximately 5 Gray of photons.

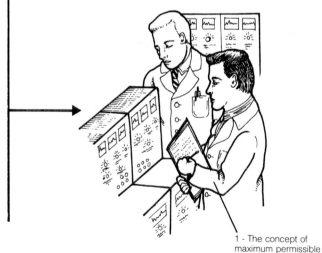

1 - Lower radiation doses causes cataract

2 - Eye

3 - Depilation occurs

4 - Testicular damage

5 - Ovarian damage

Following smaller doses of radiation (2-3 Gray), there occurs variable marrow hypoplasia which recovers, (but never to full bone marrow reserve). However, late radiation morbidity to some other tissues occurs (eg. cataracts, depilation, variable damage to testicular seminiferous epithelium or ovary). An increased risk of cancer and genetic risks occurs.

The implications of these data are many-fold. The use of nuclear weapons is detrimental to the entire human population (indeed, to all life on this planet as we know it now). The concept of maximum permissible dose and ICRP recommendations relate to low dose estimates of particularly cancer induction and genetic damage; these ICRP recommendations are expounded more fully in ICRP publications and are the guidelines for all medical radiation practice. Lastly, the

1 - The concept of maximum permissible dose is an important one

modern use of total body radiation and bone marrow transplantation for treatment of refractory leukaemias requires comment: Here the patient receives 10-12Gy (ie. above haemopoietic death) but is rescued from haemopoietic death by bone marrow transplantation. The dose of total body radiation is taken as far above the LD50 as possible without "running into" GI or lung death, (and by protracting and fractionating the dose – ie. not "flash dose" – one is able to go to 12 Gray without causing G.I. or lung death). The reason for going to a dose much higher than the LD_{50} is that one is trying to kill the last leukaemic cell.

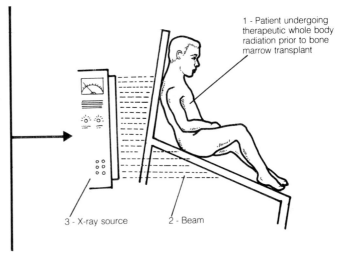

1 - Patient undergoing therapeutic whole body radiation prior to bone marrow transplant

3 - X-ray source   2 - Beam

Management of a Radioactive Leak with Human Contamination

Following the Chernobyl disaster, medical personnel should have some knowledge of management. For radio isotope leaks, contaminated clothing is immediately removed and prolonged showering/washing/scrubbing initiated without delay. Thyroid uptake of radio iodine can be blocked by the oral administration of excess stable iodine (300mg potassium iodide daily). Inhalation of particulate radio isotopes has been attempted to be recovered by pulmonary lavage.

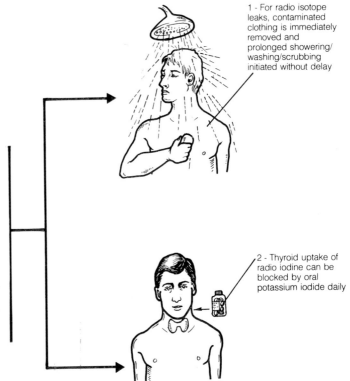

1 - For radio isotope leaks, contaminated clothing is immediately removed and prolonged showering/ washing/scrubbing initiated without delay

2 - Thyroid uptake of radio iodine can be blocked by oral potassium iodide daily

Humans receiving high radiation doses should be admitted, barrier nursed as the blood count falls, (and if it is impossible to estimate the dose they received, the depth of lymphopenia and then granulocytopenia/thrombocytopenia is useful) and supported with blood products. Following the Chernobyl disaster, the bone marrow transplant efforts were disappointing.

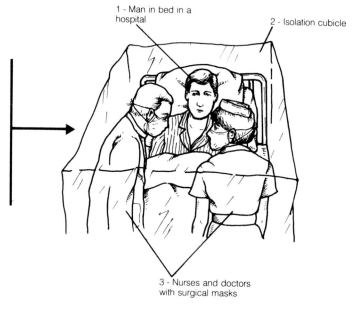

1 - Man in bed in a hospital

2 - Isolation cubicle

3 - Nurses and doctors with surgical masks

Index